THE COMPLETE GUIDE TO NATURAL HEALING OF VARICOCELE

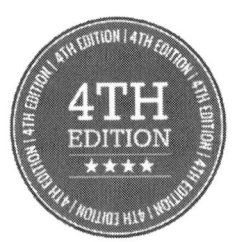

4TH EDITION

CURE PAIN, RESTORE FERTILITY,
& HEAL VARICOCELE

TOTALLY REVISED & UPDATED

DANIEL JOHNSON

Copyright © 2013-2019 Daniel Johnson

All rights reserved.

ISBN-10: 1514124459
ISBN-13: 978-1514124451

TERMS

All content, ideas, information, tips, suggestions, and concepts of this book (Content) are solely owned by the author of The Complete Guide to Natural Healing of Varicocele and Varicocele Healing Ltd (Providers). No Content may be copied, adapted, distributed, shared or transmitted without the written approval of Varicocele Healing Ltd. All rights reserved.

Anyone following this advice or ideas of this book (Reader) agrees that he/she is over 18 years of age. Reader should always consult a medical professional to determine the appropriateness of the Content. If Reader has any health problem(s) and/or concerns regarding his/her health or a medical condition, Reader should consult a medical professional as soon as possible. Never disregard medical professional advice, or delay seeking it because of Content, or anything referenced. Do not rely on Content in place of professional medical advice. If Reader develops any negative symptoms from Content, immediate discontinuation is advised. Consult a physician if the symptoms worsen or persist. If Reader has a medical emergency, immediate contact of a local medical emergency department or medical provider is advised.

Providers hold no responsibility or liability for any physical or psychological damage or for any other form of damage incurred when following any Content of this book or any referenced content. Providers neither recommend nor endorse any specific tests, products, procedures, opinions or other information that may be provided or referred to, Content is merely the viewpoint of Providers. Content is not intended nor implied to be a substitute for professional medical advice.

FOREWORD

I noticed I had a varicocele in my late teens. By this time, it had already grown to the size of a golf ball. I had no idea what it was, I went to the doctor, and she said, "Oh, that's not the biggest varicocele that I've seen." She made nothing better. Soon, I went to a surgeon to have it removed. But he didn't recommend surgery! He said it's not very effective, and there is a chance that I may lose my testicle. Surgery was not an option for me.

I was young and thought that if I'd forget about my varicocele, it would just go away. However, varicocele symptoms tend to worsen with age. It was a few years later that I could not bear the pain anymore. I also noticed that my left testicle had shrunken and become squishy. I was desperate, so I went online to seek help.

After finding generic advice like take this or that herb, I came across a book written by Bob Maloney, called "Varicocele Natural Treatment." I didn't buy into his sales pitch, but I figured that I could afford to risk $30 for a chance to recover from the constant pain and discomfort. To my surprise, a few treatments seemed like they could work! After two weeks of following his advice, I began to see results! However, his methods were incomplete.

Motivated by early results, I took matters into my own hands. I did a massive amount of research and tried many different treatments. I never got surgery, and in less than a year after beginning my treatment program, I got great results! My giant varicocele was no longer visible. I no longer experienced pain. Best of all, my shrunken and squishy left testicle grew and became plump!

You can find the treatments I used here, in The Complete Guide to Natural

Healing of Varicocele. With over 100 of the most effective natural treatments, this is the most comprehensive guide on varicocele treatment. It is the product of thorough research and proven results. In writing this guide, I studied well over 1,000 scientific publications, tested countless treatments, and used insights from my experience and education in anatomy, yoga, personal training, nutrition, health, and fitness. Most importantly, this guide has worked for thousands of others, and it is complete. After reading it, you will not need to review any other material.

Just a note on results and what to expect: This guide works. The treatments, lifestyle changes, and exercises work. I, however, understand that results vary because everyone is different, and every varicocele is caused by different risk factors. Some may follow only a few treatments and get great results, while others may need to follow many of the treatments, over a long period, to get some results. Everyone has a different set of conditions that they need to address. If you have very healthy and have been taking good care of yourself, you will probably notice results more quickly. However, if, for example, you have poor bowel health, poor posture, and high stress, you will have to work on correcting these risk factors to get good results.

So, if you get results quickly, that's great. On the other hand, if you are not noticing results, you probably have to be more patient, re-read this guide, and hone in on your personal risk factors. If you feel stuck or confused, message me, I can advise you on how to move forward.

daniel@varicocelehealing.com

CONTENTS

	Terms	iii
	Foreword	iv
1	Intro	Pg. 13
2	Cooling & Pain Relief	Pg. 31
3	Lifestyle Changes	Pg. 55
4	Fertility & Sexual Health	Pg. 65
5	Diet & Nutrition	Pg. 79
6	Fitness & Exercises	Pg. 89
7	Healing	Pg. 121
8	Fundamentals	Pg. 133
	Glossary	Pg. 139

CHAPTER 1

INTRO

SURGERY OR NATURAL TREATMENT

Look, the fact is that natural treatments and surgery are the only treatment options available for varicocele. There are no other alternatives or effective medications for varicocele treatment. And, since you are reading this book, the odds are that you do not want surgery, or are looking to enhance your surgical results.

Luckily for you, with over 100 of the best natural treatments for varicocele, The Complete Guide to Natural Healing of Varicocele is the best and most comprehensive natural treatment program for varicocele. This guide is based on thorough research and proven results. It is more effective than and safer than varicocele surgery. Follow the recommendations in this guide, and I promise you that you will notice great and risk-free results.

HOW DO NATURAL TREATMENTS WORK?

There are two premises for the treatments in this guide:

1) Lifestyle and environmental factors have a major impact on varicocele and symptom development and severity.

2) Lifestyle changes, varicocele-specific treatments, and therapeutic remedies can heal the swollen veins to a large degree, and cure varicocele

symptoms.

Notice that lifestyle changes, varicocele-specific treatments, and therapeutic remedies are all important! So, if you do not make major lifestyle changes, you will not get good results. Similarly, if you do perform varicocele-specific treatments and follow the therapeutic remedies, you will not get good results.

Be patient and persistent. Do not complain about a lack of results if you don't follow what's in the guide. And most importantly, don't judge the treatments before you give them a shot. Be patient, read through the whole guide, make the lifestyle changes, and follow the varicocele-specific treatments and therapeutic remedies. Be persistent. Sometimes it takes a bit longer to get results. If you still don't get good results after giving it a good shot, don't give up—let me know, and I will personally guide you. I am here to help get you results. Don't give up; message me!

MESSAGE ME!

Please share your experience and results with me so that I can continue to make the content better for everyone. Your feedback is important. Message me daniel@varicocelehealing.com.

OTHER TREATMENT PROGRAMS

We now offer many other treatment products and services to help maximize your treatment results. We bring a comprehensive approach to varicocele treatment that works best. Take a look at all of our treatment programs here: varicocelehealing.com/treatments.

STUD BRIEFS

Varicocele and fertility therapeutic underwear. Designed by fertility expert Dr. Spence Pentland to optimize a couple's chances of conception. Ideal for the couple that is ready to start their family or struggling to do so. Stud Briefs are essential for varicocele treatment!

TREATMENT DETAILS

+ Specially designed ultra-breathable crotch mesh maximizes cooling
+ Pushes crotch forward to further enhance cooling
+ Provides healthy scrotal support to combat sagging
+ Benefits for varicocele, fertility, & testosterone

VARACO HEALTH KIT

The Varaco Health Kit is the most effective dietary supplement for varicocele treatment. We formulated based on scientific research and on what has worked best for over 10,000 of our clients with varicocele. The Varaco Health Kit is one of our core varicocele treatment products.

TREATMENT DETAILS

+ Contains vasculoprotective properties that protect vein walls and valves
+ Helps strengthen smooth muscle lining of the veins
+ Improves vein contractility
+ Enhance varicose vein blood drainage
+ Beneficial for post-surgery complications

VARICOCELE YOGA VIDEO SERIES

Yoga is an excellent supplement for your varicocele treatment. Whether you're active or inactive, yoga brings balance to your lifestyle, helps alleviate stress, creates a healing environment, improves blood circulation, stimulates healing, and treats many varicocele risk factors.

TREATMENT DETAILS

+ 15 minute morning sequence
+ 15 minute night sequence
+ 45 minute morning sequence
+ 45 minute night sequence

PERSONALIZED TREATMENT PLAN (PTP)

Have me write you a 30 day varicocele personalized treatment plan (PTP).

For your PTP, I will first have you fill out a thorough varicocele, lifestyle, and environmental risk assessment form. I will then review your form, identify your varicocele and symptom risk factors, and develop a customized 30 day treatment plan that is most effective for you.

TREATMENT DETAILS
+ Thorough risk assessment form
+ Monthly personalized treatments
+ Unlimited Q & A
+ 1 on 1 support

FOCUS ON POSTURE

Poor posture pressurizes and swells the varicocele and aggravates the Nutcracker effect. Those who have postural problems can find it difficult even to alleviate their varicocele pain. Focus on Posture is an easy & convenient 4 minute daily workout program. This program helps strengthen the posterior chain & alleviate tightness. It helps create a body with healthy, natural, and strong alignment & mobility. Focus on Posture is especially important for you if you spend a large portion of your day sitting or in commute.

TREATMENT DETAILS
+ Easy & convenient 4 minute daily routines
+ Detailed instructions
+ Improve posture
+ Strengthen posterior chain
+ Minimize the Nutcracker Effect

PERSONAL TRAINING

Get one-on-one online coaching over Skype.

TREATMENT DETAILS
+ Varicocele specific personal training
+ Improve posture & abdominal tone
+ High stress activity risk management strategies
+ Incorporate therapeutic activities into normal workouts

+ Learn advanced training techniques

RECOMMENDED PRODUCTS

You can find a list of additional products that I recommend that we are not affiliated with Varicocele Healing here: varicocelehealing.com/more-products

WHAT IS A VARICOCELE?

Varicocele is an incidence of venous insufficiency. This means that it is the results of the failure of the veins to circulate blood. More specifically, veins have valves that prevent backward blood flow. When these valves do not close properly, blood does not circulate well, and pools. Pooled blood causes excess pressure on the vein walls, forcing them to stretch. These stretched veins are called varicose veins. More specifically, we use the term varicocele to describe the varicose veins that affect the pampiniform plexus located in the spermatic cord of the testicles.

HOW DOES VARICOCELE AFFECT YOU? WHAT ARE THE SIDE EFFECTS?

Varicocele blood pooling damages the veins and testicle. It causes vein swelling and hypersensitivity. It damages the testicles because it causes heat stress, hyper-hydration, oxidation, toxin build-up, and lack of nutrient exchange. Varicocele can cause pain, infertility, scrotal sag, testicular shrinkage, low sex drive, and impaired testosterone. Many people also experience some of the following symptoms: Embarrassment, gynecomastia, stress and anxiety, erectile dysfunction, weak or quickly lost erections, low sex drive, decreased masculinity, low motivation, decreased muscle tone, infertility, increased estrogen, and an enlarged prostate

WHAT CAUSES VARICOCELE?

Likely Not Genetically Faulty Valves

T The old and popular belief is that faulty valves cause varicocele. Faulty valves disrupt normal blood circulation, pooling blood, stretching the testicular veins, and making them varicose. However, this is a very old and outdated theory. Since then, there have been many advancements to varicocele theory.

Scientists have found many new explanations for varicocele development. These explanations mainly involve an increase in testicular vein blood pressure burden, impairment of blood circulation, toxin exposure, and impaired healing. Therefore, contrary to popular belief, varicocele is not a disorder of genetically faulty valves, it is a complex disorder. Many risk factors that cause varicocele to develop.

Do not buy into the idea that the varicocele is a genetic disorder! You are not born with malfunctioning valves. Rather, your valves function fine, but when they are excessively stressed, they begin to "malfunction." That sounds like lifestyle factors to me.

Even though we find faulty valves in about 65% of those with varicocele, we must note that this merely implies correlation and not causation. A genetic disorder is not likely to be the cause of faulty valves. Faulty valves are more a symptom of, than the cause of varicocele development.

Furthermore, scientific evidence suggests that varicocele grade and bilaterality are not heritable. The implication is that nurture factors play a critical role in the development of varicocele.

For example, a lifestyle risk factor is poor posture. Poor posture pressurizes the torso and increases blood pooling. Pooled blood causes a sixty times higher concentration of testosterone in the testicular veins. Think steroids for your testicular veins. Testosterone enlarges the testicular veins. Blood pooling also burdens the vein walls with excessive pressure, stretching the veins. Furthermore, blood pooling means the pooling of toxins and oxidizing agents that damage vein valves. Over time, this damage cause valve degeneration and malfunction.

The good news is that for most people, this is a reversible process. Treat the root cause of your varicocele! Fixing your posture will alleviate the blood pooling. It will start the process of recovery.

The Major Contributors to Varicocele Development

As mentioned earlier, many risk factors contribute to varicocele development. A major risk factor is due to the entry angle of the left spermatic vein into the left renal vein. There is a large discrepancy between the incidence of left and right-sided varicocele because the left spermatic vein drains into the left renal vein at a right angle while the right spermatic vein drains into the inferior vena cava obliquely. The right-angle entry puts excess pressure on the left spermatic vein, which in turn increases pressure on the left testicular pampiniform plexus. As well, the insertion of the left spermatic vein is 8-10 cm higher than that of the right spermatic vein, resulting in 8-10 cm greater pressure on the veins as the blood flows up through them. Increased blood pressure is the cause of varicocele development here, not faulty valves.

Another major reason for varicocele development is the nutcracker syndrome. The term nutcracker syndrome refers to how the aorta and the superior mesenteric artery compress the spermatic vein between them. This compression restricts blood flow and increases fluid pressure. The nutcracker syndrome is only present on the left side.

The nutcracker syndrome explains why those who experience bowel or digestive diseases are more likely to develop varicocele and typically experience more severe symptoms. Many bowel and digestive diseases increase inter-abdominal pressure and physically push the aorta and superior mesenteric artery together, exacerbating the nutcracker effect.

Studies have found many other risk factors for varicocele development and symptom severity. These factors include but are not limited to: Obesity, overweight, stress, physical trauma, height (taller is worse), testicular dysfunction, high Nitric Oxide expression in the spermatic cord, posterior nutcracker syndrome, scrotal sag, chronic cough, constipation, bowel problems (e.g. irritable bowel syndrome and inflammatory bowel disease), abdominal bloating, weak or hyperactive pelvic floor muscle, stress, improper lymph drainage, improper nutrition, lack of exercise, prolonged sitting, long-distance running and biking, high exertion during exercise, jumping activities (e.g. basketball and volleyball), postural imbalances, and prolonged standing. Notice how most of these factors either impair blood flow or increase blood pressure in the pampiniform plexus.

Some rare medical conditions may also cause the development of a varicocele. I recommend consulting a qualified medical practitioner, just in case. These conditions include renal cell carcinoma (tumor), retroperitoneal tumor, retroperitoneal fibrosis, and liver cirrhosis (caused by portal hypertension). These are rare cases, but do not rule them out without professional medical clearance.

HOW IS VARICOCELE DIAGNOSED?

Due to advances in diagnostic techniques, the current belief is that varicocele may affect as much as 20% of men. Varicocele diagnostic criteria fall under four categories: Subclinical, grade I, grade II, and grade III.

Subclinical: Ultrasound analysis but not physical exam detects the presence of a varicocele.

Note that, a subclinical varicocele can still cause severe symptoms, even though higher grades typically cause more severe symptoms. This is because blood reflux can be present without the presence of swelling.

Grade I: The varicocele is only palpable during or after Valsalva maneuver.

Grade II: The varicocele is palpable without Valsalva maneuver.

Grade III: The varicocele is visible through the skin to the eyes (seen as a lump or "bag of worms").

WHY THIS GUIDE?

This is The Complete Guide to Natural Healing of Varicocele. No guide like it exists. It is the result of thorough research and proven results. It has information from over 1,000 scientific publications. There are over 100 different treatments in this guide. Every treatment comes with details on its anatomical significance, and instructions on how to perform it effectively. It is the most comprehensive guide on natural varicocele treatment. By reading this guide, you will know more about varicocele and varicocele treatment than most physicians! After reading this guide, you will not need to review any other material. It is complete.

I highly recommend reading the guide in its entirety to get a full understanding of the multidimensionality of varicocele and aid you in better understanding how to select the treatments that are most effective and relevant to your case. To heal your varicocele and to prevent its reoccurrence, you must perform some corrective therapy, and make lifestyle changes. The good news is that most lifestyle changes are easy to make and accompany with them many other positive life-improving benefits.

THIS IS THE RIGHT GUIDE FOR YOU IF YOU WANT TO:
- ✓ Reduce Varicocele Size
- ✓ Undo Testicular Shrinkage
- ✓ Alleviate Pain
- ✓ Reduce Scrotal Sag
- ✓ Improve Fertility
- ✓ Increase Testosterone & Normalize Hormones
- ✓ Enhance Sexual Performance
- ✓ Attain Pre- or Post-Surgery Enhancement

Reduce Varicocele Size

Healing your varicocele involves reducing venous pressure, creating an ideal healing environment, stimulating the healing and strengthening of damaged tissue, and providing proper nutrients that will stimulate the improvement of venous tone.

Ever ask yourself why so many people only develop varicose veins next to their testicles? Well, there are several anatomical reasons why. Caring for them will do wonders for the healing of your varicocele.

The healing process requires the removal of stress factors and the provision of a more nurturing environment for your veins. Healing is the point of this guide, and actually, all treatment methods presented are relevant to it. Read the entire guide! You never know, one treatment may make all the difference for you.

Undo Testicular Shrinkage

Blood pooling causes damage to the testicle on the affected side. It deprives the testis of nutrients, exposes it to excess toxins, and creates heat stress. In time, testicular shrinkage follows. However, testicular shrinkage usually occurs on both sides because damage to one testicle disrupts normal testosterone production. In healthy individuals, testosterone is responsible for the growth and development of both testicles.

Decreased testicular volumes of 43%, 53%, and 73% occur in individuals with varicocele grades I, II, and III, respectively.

Most of the treatments in this book aim to minimize blood pooling, and stimulating both testicular healing and growth.

Alleviate Pain
Aching or pain arises from the testicles and varicocele. Furthermore, both short and long-term stressors can cause pain.

Short-term pain is short-lasting (hours to days) and may be caused by:

1) Heavy blood pooling and little drainage for prolonged periods
2) Prolonged heat stress
3) Physical stress (e.g., from penis enlargement exercises or biking)
4) Blood toxicity
5) Etc.

Long-term pain can be felt for up to weeks and is typically caused by:

1) Years of bad habits (lifestyle changes are required)
2) Unhealthy testicles (e.g., due to genital heat stress or toxicity)
3) Excess body weight
4) Chronic constipation or improper digestion/bowel movements
5) Etc.

This guide has specific remedies for curing both short and long-term pain, though all of the remedies should help alleviate pain to some degree.

Reduce Scrotal Sag
The testicles need to be 1-3°C/2-5°F below normal body temperature to function correctly. That is why they are outside of the body in the scrotum, which effectively regulates their temperature. The scrotum sags away from the body to cool the testicles and tightens to warm them.

However, contrary to popular belief, scrotal sagging is not the major cooling mechanism of the testicles. The major cooling mechanism of the testicles is the counter current cooling effect of the pampiniform plexus. The pampiniform plexus is a meshwork of veins that run counter to arteries that carry warm blood from the heart. This meshwork absorbs the warm arterial blood and cooling it, before it reaches the testicles. Varicocele is enlargement of the pampiniform plexus, and therefore abolishes the counter current cooling mechanism of the testicles. Thus, the scrotum constantly hangs low since it cannot alleviate the heat.

Scrotal sagging also occurs because varicocele weighs down the scrotum. Over years, the weighing down causes the tissues that keep the scrotum tight against the body to loosen and the skin and connective tissues to stretch. Thus, the affected testicle hangs lower and lower.

This guide has treatments for improving scrotal muscle tone and blood circulation, as well as treatments for cooling the testicles without damaging them.

Improve Fertility

About one-fourth to one-third of men diagnosed with varicocele experience fertility problems. That is about 5-8% of all men! Parameters used to assess male fertility include sperm count, volume, morphology, and motility, as well as sperm DNA damage and testicular volume. Typically, at least several of these parameters are negatively affected in those with varicocele.

It is not abnormal for varicocele severity, and fertility worsen with age. Therefore, it is essential to stop the disease or mitigate its negative effects as soon as possible.

There are an endless number of ways improve your fertility and chances of a successful pregnancy, many of which are beyond the scope of this book.

The varicocele healing guide includes treatments to improve testicular health and function, and protect the sperm tail, head and DNA against varicocele toxic blood pooling.

Increase Testosterone & Normalize Hormones

Varicocele disrupts normal testosterone production. This causes an array of negative symptoms, including gynecomastia (enlargement of male breast tissue), erectile dysfunction, lower sex drive, decreased masculinity, low motivation, testicular shrinkage, lower muscle tone, excess fat, and more.

Luckily, normalizing hormone levels, as long as your varicocele has not progressed too far is relatively easy and the negative symptoms (with partial exception to few) are reversible by restoring normal hormone balance.

Normalizing hormone levels is a bi-product of most of the treatments in this book. However, for completeness purposes, I have provided some specific treatments for it as well.

Enhance Sexual Performance

Erectile dysfunction, weak or easily lost erections, and poor sexual performance are all associated with varicocele.

Again, luckily correcting this is relatively easy (similar to normalizing hormones); the results will come as you follow the treatments outlined in this guide. A few treatments targeting sexual performance are also provided for completeness purposes.

Pre- & Post-Surgery Enhancement

Surgery is not a very effective treatment for varicocele and comes with serious risks. Aside from the possibility of losing a testicle, the fact is that you are cutting out (ligating) the varicose veins. So, fewer veins are spared to uptake blood circulation, and there is an increased burden on the remaining veins. There is also the possibility of getting scar tissue from the incision. Varicocele can also redevelop in up to 20% of cases. Often, there is no testicular hypertrophy (regaining of lost testicular size) and normal fertility does not resume 86% of the time. As well, varicocele surgery is neither effective nor recommended for the treatment of pain. As a matter of fact, surgery may not be effective at all, and is one of the most controversial topics in the field of andrology.

Embolization, in my opinion, is a quick and dirty alternative to surgery. It uses metal coils to try and target the varicose veins. It is generally less effective than surgery. It also has many associated risks and a much higher rate of hydrocele formation. And, do you really want metal coils in your testicular veins for the rest of your life?

Do you want to understand varicocele better? Do you want to know what to do to reduce the chances of varicocele redeveloping post-surgery? Do you want to stimulate testicular growth and normalize fertility? This book is the best place to go for a complete guide for what to do and not to do when it comes to caring for your testicles and vein health.

QUICK OVERVIEW OF THE HEALING GUIDE

There are eight chapters in this book. The chapters are not in any particular order. The following is a quick overview of the book's chapters:

Chapter 2: Cooling & Pain Relief

Keeping your testicles cool is the first step in the healing process. You cannot induce healing when your testicles are suffering from genital heat stress. There are right and wrong ways of cooling, and I address both in this chapter.

When it comes to pain relief, think: Cool, circulate, and stimulate healing.

Chapter 3: Lifestyle Changes

There are many lifestyle changes that you can make will make a significant positive impact on the state of your varicocele, and your fertility. This chapter contains the many things you should do and should avoid doing during the healing process.

Chapter 4: Fertility & Sexual Health

Do you want plump testicles, rock hard erections, high testosterone levels, and to increase your sperm count and ejaculate volume? The treatments in this chapter are select to improve all these, and at the same time aid in the healing process.

Chapter 5: Diet & Nutrition

This chapter focuses on the dietary changes and supplements that will make the most significant impact on improving the status of your varicocele, and in aiding your treatment process.

Chapter 6: Fitness & Exercises
This chapter is essential because it teaches the specific exercises that you need to do to reduce excess pressure that causes varicocele. I teach how to zero the risk of exercising and activity on varicocele. Moreover, I have also compiled the best yoga and tai-chi exercises for treating varicocele risk factors.

Chapter 7: Healing
This chapter contains treatments that are essential for varicocele healing. Note: Do not neglect the other chapters, as they are necessary for reducing varicocele and treating your symptoms.

Chapter 8: The Fundamentals
This chapter contains a set of the most effective varicocele treatments that you need to follow! Note: You still have to read through the entire guide to identify your personal risk factors.

HOW LONG DOES HEALING TAKE?
How long will healing take? Well, that depends on which variable you are considering. Just keep in mind that the best results come with time. You cannot build Michelangelo's David in one day, neither can you fix years of bad habits in a month. However, you can be well on your way to greatness in a month. Take your time. There is no rush. View Table 1 to see how long you should expect healing to take if you follow this guide.

Treatment Variable	Minimum	Maximum
Short Term Pain	5 min	7 days
Long Term Pain	7 days	3 months
Subclinical Varicocele	1 month	4 months
Grade I Varicocele	2 months	6 months
Grade II Varicocele	3 months	8 months
Grade III Varicocele	4 months	1 year
Scrotal Sag	1 month	4 months
Testicular Shrinkage	2 months	8 months
Infertility	2 months	1 year

Table 1: Presents the minimum and maximum time it takes to treat each treatment variable. Note: Treatment duration typically depends on the severity of the disease. Higher grade varicoceles take longer to treat than minor cases. Treatment duration time also depends on treatment compliance and the amount of effort that you put into your recovery. Note: This is not to say that you have to follow all the treatment methods in this book. Instead, focus on finding the treatments that work best for you and your lifestyle.

Most people who consistently follow this guide notice some improvement in as little as three days to a week! Now, your results may appear to come and go for the first few months. Results come and go in part because of inconsistency with your lifestyle changes and treatment compliance. As well, because some activities (e.g., strenuous exercise, chain-smoking, sitting for 12 hours a day, stomach acidity, etc.) can impair the healing process and re-damage the veins and testicles. So, it is essential to stay consistent. Focus on the long-term process of healing. Consider the short-term results that come and go as indicators that you are on the right track. Keep going! Your results will become more and more consistent with time.

Varicocele and symptom severity, as well as your treatment compliance, will determine how long your healing process will take. The most effective approach is to find the treatments that are most important for you and follow them religiously!

You can also opt to follow the simple lifestyle changes and easy-to-follow treatments. Doing so can minimize the time you spend on varicocele treatment. It can reduce any related stress that you may have. And, really, help you continue the long-term process that is necessary for healing. From there, one day, not today, not tomorrow, but a few months down the road, you will look down in the mirror and notice amazing results.

CHAPTER DEFINITIONS

Arteries: Carry oxygenated blood (from lungs to heart and from the heart to bodily tissues)

Grade I Varicocele: Grade 1 varicocele is only palpable during Valsalva maneuver.

Grade II Varicocele: Grade 2 varicocele is palpable without Valsalva maneuver.

Grade III Varicocele: Grade 3 varicocele is normally visible through the skin (seen as a lump or "bag of worms").

Pampiniform Plexus (Veins): Veins that drain from the testicles. They also function to cool the testicles.

Reflux: Backflow (flow in the wrong direction) of blood.

Subclinical Varicocele: Ultrasound analysis but not physical exam detects the presence of a subclinical varicocele.

Testis: (Singular) one testicle.

Varicocele: Enlarged testicular veins. More specifically, it refers to the enlargement of the pampiniform plexus (veins).

Valves: Veins have one directional valves that prevent blood from flowing backwards and circulating in one direction.

Varicose Veins: Enlarged veins (general).

Veins: Carry de-oxygenated blood (from heart to lungs and from bodily tissues back to heart).

Venous Insufficiency: Inability for veins to circulate blood.

DANIEL JOHNSON

CHAPTER 2

COOLING & PAIN RELIEF

PAIN & HEAT STRESS

What Causes Varicocele Pain

Why does varicocele cause pain? The simple answer is blood pooling, heat damage, and stress. So, if you reduce blood pooling, cool your testicles, and alleviate the stressors, you should be able to relieve your pain quickly. However, this chapter is further simplified, stating that pain relief is achieved by cooling and circulating. To learn how to alleviate the stressors, please make sure to read the rest of the book.

As explained in the intro, the spermatic veins that leave the testicles form a meshwork of veins called the pampiniform plexus. The pampiniform plexus encircle the arteries that bring blood to the testicles. These create a counter-current heat exchange mechanism that cools the warm arterial blood going to the testicles. Varicocele effectively abolishes this mechanism, causing elevated scrotal temperatures. Higher temperatures increase metabolic activity, deplete nutrients, cause oxidative and hypotonic stress, and come with a whole array of other factors that result in testicular damage.

Sperm concentration, motility, and testosterone production deteriorate with the with elevated average daily scrotal temperatures. These are irrespective of varicocele grade. High temperatures have a negative impact partially because the testicles have enzymes and structures that are only effective at lower temperatures. These enzymes and structures function optimally at 1-3°C/2-5°F below normal body temperature (normal body temperature is

37°C/98.5°F). Moreover, higher temperatures increase metabolic rate, and can destabilize testicular and sperm structures.

The severity of varicocele typically increases with age and results in an increase in the rate of damage through positive feedback mechanisms. This is why, even though most people do not experience pain early on in their disease, they begin to have more regular and intense pain as their varicocele progresses.

Pain attributed to the testicles is very common. This pain occurs during exposure of the testicles to excess stress (i.e., excess heat, poor blood flow, low nutrients, etc.) throughout the day or over longer periods. So, the best thing to do is remove the stressors, normalize blood flow, and rest to allow recovery. Next time prevent or minimize the stressor to not cause any pain in the first place.

Pain can also originate from the varicose veins. This type of pain occurs when enlarged varicose veins are tugged around, squeezed tight, or exposed to excess pressure and toxin build-up. It can also be due to micro-trauma (e.g., from the bike seat). The sensation normally comes directly from the veins but can also arise from tissue surrounding the veins (including the testis).

Cooling for Pain Relief

The problem is that we cannot avoid unnatural sources of heat with our modern lifestyle. So, both cooling treatments and heat risk management are essential.

Scientific studies have proven that cooling treatments alone are enough to help alleviate pain symptoms and significantly improve semen quality in about 70% of men! Cooling can also help boost testosterone. There are many daily heat risk factors that we must manage. Think of it as restoring optimal testicular function! If you want plump testicles, cool your balls!

HOW DO YOU CHECK FOR NORMAL TESTICULAR TEMPERATURE?

You should note that "normal" testicular temperature fluctuates throughout the day. It is natural and healthy. Focus on keeping your testicles cool on average, not 100% of the time. Your goal is to normalize testicular temperature and prevent heat stress, not to constantly and always keep your testicles cool.

Method 1: Hand on Thighs, Then Touch
Place the palm of your hands on your thighs for 20 seconds and then touch your testicles. Normal testicular temperature should feel lightly cool to the touch. This is a relatively accurate way of estimating testicular temperature—without using a thermometer.

Method 2: Circulate, Then Touch
Perform an inversion for 5-10 minutes (e.g., legs up on the wall, or bridge pose, or by just elevating your hips with a pillow while lying down). Make sure to allow adequate heat ventilation. After the inversion, touch your testicles to feel what normal testicular temperature feels like. Compare this to your testicular temperature when you're wearing clothes, sitting down, or exercising.

Method 3: Touch Often
Once you figure out what normal testicular temperature feels like, you should feel your testicles multiple times a day, for a few weeks. Just learn when they are too hot and when they are at a normal temperature. Don't just assume! It's hard to guess when your testicles are overheated. It is critical to feel your testicles often. Learn when they are overheated and start to take corrective action.

Method 4: Scrotal Sag
Scrotal sag is not the most accurate way of figuring out normal testicular temperature. Sagging typically means that your testicles are too hot, and your body is trying to cool them by distancing them from your body. Note that your scrotum naturally tightens up and relaxes throughout the day. Do not worry about it. This is natural and healthy. It simply means that the scrotal sag is not very accurate indicator. So, if you can, feel your testicles instead.

Cautionary Note
Just a cautionary note for when you perform these treatments: Do not

over-cool your testicles. 37°C/98.5°F is your normal body temperature. 34-36°C/93.5-96.5°F is an ideal temperature of your testicles. It is only 1-3°C/2-5°F lower than your normal body temperature! Your goal is to normalize, not to cause testicular hypothermia!

On the other hand, temporary changes in temperature are okay! It is not a big deal to get into a hot tub, over-cool your testicles, or take a hot shower—once in a while. Your testicles are not delicate snowflakes. Your goal is to keep your testicles at a normal temperature in general, not 24/7. I cannot emphasize enough that your goal is long-term prevention, and not short-term worry and self-stress.

QUICK COOLING & PAIN RELIEF

Whenever you experience varicocele pain, you should take a mental note of what you think caused you to experience the pain. Maybe you were wearing tight underwear all day, exercised with pants and underwear that over-heated your testicles, were very constipated that day, masturbated excessively over the past few days, etc. Figure out what might have caused the pain, and try to avoid it. Of course, you may just have chronic pain from long-term damage—this needs time to heal and recover.

In any case, this section relevant if you want to minimize both acute and chronic pain quickly.

Cool, Circulate & Rest

The best and quickest way for most people to alleviate their varicocele pain is to perform a cooling treatment, inversion, and then rest. Cooling treatments could include a cool shower, pointing a fan toward your crotch, applying a cooling pack, etc. Inversions are any positions where your hips are above your torso, including feet up on the wall, shoulder stand, bridge pose, etc. Resting includes be lying down, meditation, napping, sleep, etc.

Lay Down

Being vertical (e.g., standing or sitting) builds up a lot of pressure in your varicocele. Blood has to move vertically up against the force of gravity, from the scrotum to the heart. Being horizontal (e.g., lying down) in general decreases your blood pressure because your heart does not have to pump blood against the force of gravity. Similarly, this is why varicocele swelling reduces when lying down.

Lying down is good enough to drain pooled blood, improve circulation, and cool down your testicles. It is a great way to drain your varicocele, and quickly cool and relieve stressful pressure that could be causing pain. To allow your testicles to cool down adequately, lay down without pants and underwear. Note that being relaxed and stress-free is healthier and better than freezing your entire body just to cool your testicles.

Just a further note, lying down is also a good way of relaxing and changing the gravitational directional pull on your digestive tract. It helps to pass gas and can stimulate a bowel movement. Gas passage and bowel movements decrease bloating and abdominal pressure (good for reducing varicocele swelling). When lying down, you can further stimulate gas passage and bowel movements by rolling around and stretching.

Napping

If you are experiencing pain or your testicles are not feeling optimal, napping is a great way of helping them recover. Again, since you are lying down horizontally when you sleep, your blood pressure is much lower. In contrast to lying down, napping also stimulates healing, helps decrease inflammation, and drops the body's temperature by about 1°C/2°F, all of which are good for pain relief and recovery.

It is generally true that varicocele swelling and symptoms are lowest when waking up in the morning and worsen as the day progresses. Napping is, therefore, a great way to re-set things to the waking state.

I recommend sleeping bottomless when possible. At most, only wear loose-fitting underwear or just thin pajamas—without underwear. You can wear as much as you like on your upper and lower body, but let your hips and testicles get some air!

Legs up on Wall

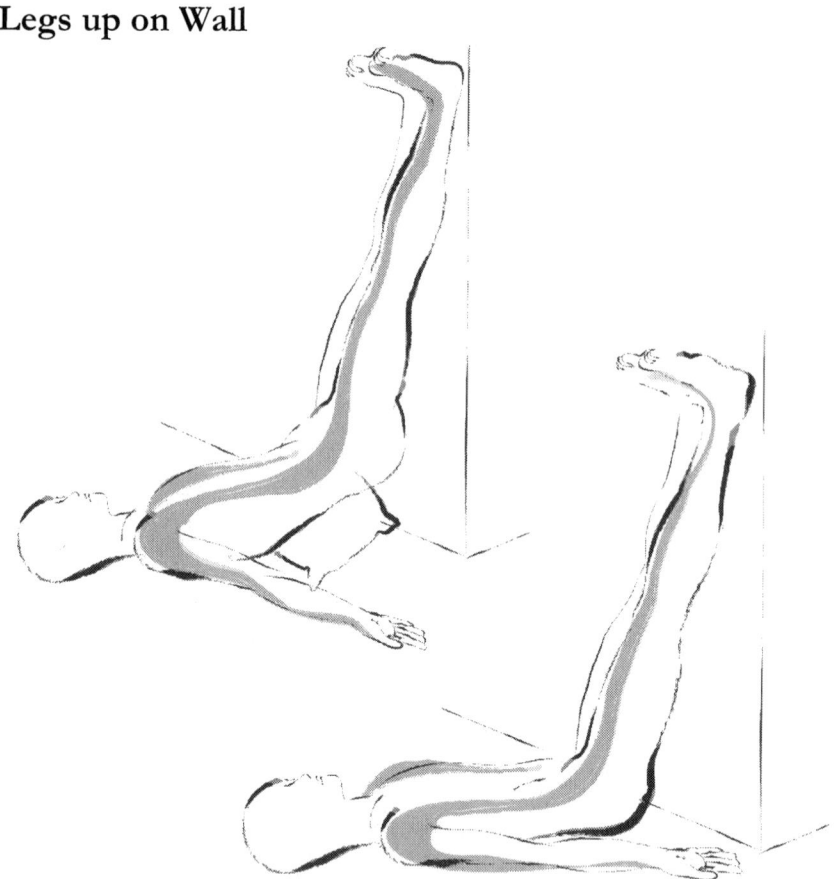

When lying down is not enough to drain or cool your varicocele, you can perform an inversion! Inversions elevate the pelvis above the heat, draining pooled blood and improving blood circulation to cool the testicles. Inversions work because varicocele is not a problem of the arteries, but of the veins that travel from the pelvis back to the heart. So, turning upside down (inverting) allows blood more easily flow back to the heart, with the aid of gravity.

If anything, only remember this one exercise! It is my favorite. It is the easiest and best pose for long-term healing (helps cool & circulate). It is great for quick cooling and pain relief. It is also easy to hold for a time, so I consider it better than the bridge pose. I can't emphasize enough how helpful it is to keep your feet up on the wall for a long time! It is also super important because when your varicocele is drained, you can perform treatments that would have otherwise been high risk to perform (discussed later in the guide).

Inversions have the added benefit of naturally normalizing testicular temperature. That is because inversions work by draining the varicocele and normalizing blood circulation. Therefore, because normal blood circulation allows the counter current heat exchange mechanism of the testicles to work properly, your testicles will naturally approach their optimal temperature. This means that you do not have to worry about over-cooling or over-heating your testicles when performing inversions.

To perform this pose, simply put your legs up on a wall. You can enhance this pose by propping your hips up with a pillow.

Legs up on the wall pose is ideal at night in bed, before sleeping. It is a relaxing exercise, so it can help you fall asleep better too. You can also put a blanket over yourself while mid-inversion, and maybe fall asleep after.

You can also perform this pose at the gym or anywhere in the house—all you need is the floor, maybe a mat, and a wall!

Early in your treatment, I recommend performing this exercise every day for at least 5-10 minutes. Perform it 1-2 times per day, or as many times as you like.

Cold Water Treatment

Cold water treatments can be very beneficial for both your veins and testicles. Cold constricts veins. It helps tone the smooth muscle lining of your varicocele. It is anti-inflammatory. It pulls makes the scrotum pull up and makes the scrotum tight. It helps flush out varicocele toxic blood pooling. It cools down overheated testicles and allows them to function better. Cold water treatments are very effective for healing varicocele, treating varicocele pain, and improving both fertility and testosterone. It is essential for varicocele treatment.

Perform a cold water treatment before exercising, after sitting for long periods, on hot days, after prolonged scrotal heat stress, and even after physical damage to the testicles to testicular veins (e.g., from biking, or/acute injuries, etc.)

water over your testicles for 10-15 seconds; repeat 2-5 times. Take 10-15 seconds breaks in between sets. Perform this ideally 1 time per day, and up to 3 times if needed.

Cautionary note: Be aware that you can also over-cool your testicles. Do not perform a cold water treatment for prolonged periods (e.g. longer than 15 seconds). The general rule of thumb is: If it feels okay on your face, it's okay on your balls!

Cool to Cold Shower

Cold showers are amazingly beneficial for varicocele, fertility, and testosterone. Taking a cold shower, over your entire body, is a great way to cool down the testicles, strongly activate the cremaster reflex, get great anti-inflammatory benefits, improve the immune system, massively boost testosterone, and enhance the body's healing capacity! Cold showers are a great habit to develop for men with varicocele.

An important benefit of a cold shower, that's further noteworthy, is its strong effect on toning the cremaster muscle (the smooth muscle lining your scrotum). The side affected by varicocele usually hangs lower. Varicocele weighs down, and over time loosen up the cremaster muscle. Hanging increases the volume of blood that pools! Therefore, strengthening your cremaster muscle will tuck up on your varicocele and naturally reduce its size. Strengthening the cremaster muscle is critical for long-term healing.

Cold showers are also essential after a long day of work, post-exercise, and after excessive heat exposure. They are also an excellent routine for waking up in the mornings.

Here is how you can start: Make it a long-term goal! For the first few weeks, start with hot water, and then slowly cool it down to a bearable point. Bearable means that you are not uncomfortable!

Then upgrade: Start with only warm water, and then slowly cool down to a slightly uncomfortable point.

Upgrade further: Start with lukewarm water, and then slowly cool down to the same, slightly uncomfortable point.

Slowly, over a year, work your way up to starting with cool to cold water, and ending with very cold water! Take your time; be patient. Always make it bearable and feel good!

You can even play around with it like this: The colder the water is, the shorter the treatment duration. For example, if you use water that's just lightly cool, you can bear it for 3-5 minutes with ease. However, as you use colder and colder water, you can reduce the duration of your treatment to even 5-15 seconds. Slowly, work your way up to colder temperatures and longer durations.

Caution: The point is not to give yourself hypothermia. Technically, even the very cold showers should be bearably uncomfortable, and actually feel good! You are not trying to hurt yourself--you are performing a therapeutic treatment.

DAYTIME

Proper Pants

Now I know the odds are that no one told you, but tight-fitting pants are bad because they constrict natural blood circulation and put unnecessary pressure on your body. Ideally, you should wear breathable and well-fitted pants. Your pants should not be tight around your hips or waist. They should have a light and comfortable feel and fit.

The same thing applies to any belts! Do not make your belt excessively tight around your waist! Give your blood and bowels space to flow.

If your pants are too tight, you can stretch them out, get them fitted, cut them loose, or just throw them out. Buying new and healthier pants is well worth the investment.

Proper Underwear

Proper underwear can be a great therapeutic tool for both pain relief and long-term healing. Bellow, I summarize the properties of therapeutic underwear.

Breathes Well: Pretty self-explanatory, but critically important. If the underwear breathes well, it is good. If not, then do not wear it. Both fabric type and thickness matter. I have read that cotton transfers heat best, but that is not true at all. I prefer polyester type fabrics and fabric that are both thin and designed to transfer heat like Nike's Dryfit, and Adidas' Climacool boxer briefs. But it is okay if you find any other fabric type that also breathes well or is meant for cooling.

Remember how I said to feel your testicles a few times a day? Well, that's how you know if your underwear breathes well. If you feel your testicles, and they are often hot, then your underwear does not breathe well. Your testicles should be at their normal temperature throughout the day.

Provides Scrotal Support: Light scrotal support can help reduce scrotal sag and blood pooling. This is helpful in the long-run for minimizing symptoms and improving healing. Light scrotal support means that the fabric gently supports your testicles.

Note that a little additional support can be helpful for strenuous activities (e.g. heavy lifting, weightlifting, basketball, martial arts, etc.)

Also note that if you have to choose either underwear that breathes well or underwear that provides support, I recommend picking the underwear that breathes well 100% of the time.

Improper Underwear

Improper underwear can cause aches, pains, infertility, and worsen varicocele severity. I cannot emphasize how much of a difference the underwear you wear makes on your symptoms.

Overheats Testicles: Overheating the testicles increases blood pooling, causes aches and pains, halts sperm production, destroys testosterone levels, and increases varicocele severity. I do not mean to sound overly dramatic, but testicular hyperthermia is very underrated. Avoid underwear that traps heat or has thick or excess fabric. Again, you will have to touch your testicles and check several times throughout the day to see if your underwear overheats your testicles or not.

Too Tight Around Scrotum: Underwear that is tight around the scrotum physically irritates the testicles, prevents testicular self-thermoregulation by physically stopping them from dropping down to cool (the cremaster reflex), and tends to over-heat the testicles. Typically, negative symptoms show within a few hours of wearing underwear that is too tight around the scrotum. Go for light support, not compression.

Too Tight Around the Waist: Same as wearing tight pants or a tight belt, underwear that is too tight around your waist increases intra-abdominal pressure and makes it difficult for blood to circulate. I highly recommend getting well-fitted underwear.

Underwear Types

Going Commando: If your underwear is causing you bad symptoms, I recommend going commando (without any underwear), until you get better underwear. Going commando is good because it helps keep your testicles cool, is bad because does not provide support.

Wet Underwear: Making your underwear wet with some water is a good method of enhancing their thermo-conductivity. This is a great tip/trick for when going to the gym, a run, bike ride, or any other physical activity.

Boxers: Boxers are typically better for heat transfer, however, they provide no support.

Boxer Briefs: Boxer briefs are better for support, however, they typically trap more heat. Some boxer briefs are too tight around the scrotum.

Jockstraps: Jockstraps typically provide good scrotal support, however at times they can be too tight. Thinner jockstraps allow better testicular thermo-regulation.

Fertility Underwear: Fertility underwear is probably your best bet for getting all of the good and none of the bad out of your underwear. Fertility underwear typically has good thermo-conductivity and provides good support. However, you need to do research to get the best product, and typically have to pay a premium (high cost) for them.

Beware the Cushiony Chair

Cushiony chairs trap heat and have been shown elevate scrotal temperature by 3-4°C/5-7°F! Saddle chairs are more ideal but less comfortable. Try to avoid cushiony chairs when you can, whether at home, in the car, or at work. However, if you do sit on cushiony chairs, you should try some of the following: Be comfortable—but sit more with your legs spread than crossed. Get up occasionally to allow the heat to dissipate. Point a fan toward your crotch (or in your direction) to improve circulation. Put an ice pack near your crotch to keep the general area cool. If you are at home, use the circle-cut pants (see later in this chapter), or just go pantless and/or underwearless. You can also sit at the edge of your chair, improving both your sitting posture and heat ventilation.

Proper Sitting Techniques

Excessive sitting is the new smoking. Actually, it is much worse than smoking. It is as bad as smoking, drinking and having diabetes. Sitting all day is a big contributing factor to varicocele development and severity. It leads to poor posture, core deactivation, muscular and postural imbalances, elevates scrotal temperature, and impairs breathing, blood circulation, and bowel movements.

Now, I know most of us have to sit for travel, work, and entertainment. So, here are some great tips if you do have to sit:

Arm Rests: When possible use the arm rests (note that this is not necessarily good for posture in the long-run.

Avoid Tight Pants and Belts: Tight pants and belts really exacerbate the negative effects of sitting. They tighten and pressurize the torso, and prevent proper breathing, digestion, and blood circulation. If you are wearing a tight belt, loosen it up a notch. Ideally, wear well fitted pants or ones that have stretchable/flexible waists.

Belly Breathing: Belly breathing when sitting will help improve blood and lymph circulation, aid in digestion and bowel movement, and help bring better awareness to the stressors on the torso.

Consider Investing in Better Technology: If you regularly sit for long periods, seriously consider investing in a standing desk, ergonomic chair, monitor/screen elevating mount/platform, personal trainer, physiotherapist, posture brace, etc.

Footrest: Putting your legs up on a footrest helps reduce varicocele swelling and decrease blood pressure.

Lean Against the Back Rest: Instead of all your weight weighing down on your torso, you can lean back and let the back rest of the chair take some of your weight. You can also improve this effect by lightly pushing yourself back into the seat by pushing your feet forward.

Lean Back with Your Hips Forward: Leaning back with your hips forward is not always convenient or possible, but it can reduce the pressure in your torso/testicular veins.

Lower Abdominal Tuck: Do not allow your lower abdomen to protrude/sag out excessively. Sometimes, keep it tight, flexed and pulled in. Try this for a portion of the time you spend setting. It will make a big difference.

Posture 1: Spinal Alignment: Good sitting posture starts with spinal alignment. The idea is to retain normal spinal alignment even when sitting. So, when possible, start by tilting your hips forward to attain normal lumbar (lower back) alignment. Then raise your chest up to attain normal thoracic (torso) alignment. Lastly pull your shoulders down and back, and then tuck your chin in and pull your head back to attain normal cervical (neck) alignment.

Posture 2: Adjust Your Screen Height: The higher your screen is, the easier it is for you to align your torso and head /neck. This means less forward lean and less pressure on the torso/testicular veins.

Posture 3: Tilt Seat Forward: Tilting your seat forward brings the lower back (lumbar spine) into better alignment. Lower back alignment allows for better overall posture/spinal alignment.

Posture 4: Sit at the Edge of Your Seat: Sitting at the edge of your seat tilts your hips forward, creating better lower back (lumbar spine) alignment, and allowing better posture. Sitting at the edge of your seat also has the added benefit of improving heat transfer to the testicles, and therefore should be commonly practiced.

Proper Heat Transfer: Keep legs spread apart, change sitting position regularly, lift butt off seat for a moment, sit at the edge of your seat, wear thinner pants/underwear, get up for regular breaks, etc.

Resting Posture: You cannot sit with perfect posture all day. Therefore it is good to know a few good relaxed positions that you can rely on when tired, for example: Lean against the back of your seat, lean back at an angle with your hips forward, lean your head/torso onto the table, rest your arms on the arm rest/table, lean forward onto the table and hold your weight up with your arms, etc.

Take Breaks: Do not sit for prolonged periods (more than two hours) without getting up to take a break, stand, move, and stretch.

The Sitting Ideal: Ideally, you want to combine as many of the outlined proper sitting techniques as possible. For example, lean back against the back rest of the chair, sit with good posture, spread your legs apart, perform abdominal breathing (not mentioned here), and ensure good heat transfer.

Counteracting the Negative Effects of Sitting

If you sit (or used to sit) for prolonged periods, there are several things that you need to do to counteract the negative effects. Think: Stretch, strengthen, realign, activity, and breaks.

Be Active: Sitting is a form of inactivity. Therefore, if you sit for prolonged periods, you need to make sure you perform both light and high intensity activities regularly. It also helps to be active before and after sitting to help stimulate muscular activity (e.g. for posture).

Spinal Realignment (Advanced): Perform lumbar, thoracic and cervical realignment techniques.

Strengthen (Advanced): Strengthen your hip flexors, quadriceps, posterior chain (hamstrings, glutes, spinal erectors, and back muscles), shoulder depressors, shoulder external rotators, hyoid muscles and cervical extensors.

Stretch (Advanced): Stretch your hip flexors, hamstrings, and shoulder elevators and internal rotators.

Take Breaks: Try not to sit for long periods without a break. A good rule to follow is for every hour of sitting, take a 5 minute active break.

Travel

I have had a lot of people ask me about long-distance travel. If you are experiencing varicocele discomfort or pain during long-distance travel, you have to figure out what is specifically affecting you. Are your testicles overheated and damaged? Are you wearing tight pants or underwear? Are your testicles overheating during travel? Do you have digestive or postural issues that could worsen your symptoms? Do you masturbate before travel? Is the cushiony chair in your car trapping a lot of heat (if so, maybe invest in a better over-lay)? Is your core overly inactive during travel (if so, perform a lower-abdominal for a portion of your travel time)?

The recommendations are the same as the other recommendations in this guide. Just figure out how to cool, circulate, and minimize stressors.

If you sit for long periods, make sure to refer to the Proper Sitting Technique section earlier in this chapter.

Laptop on Legs

This one should go without explaining. A Laptop can heat up—a lot! You do not want to spend hours with it on your lap. If you are going to place a laptop on your lap, place something in between the laptop and your lap, preferably something hard that does not transfer heat.

SLEEPING

Sleeping is a great time for healing! Everyone sleeps, so there is no excuse for not making your sleep therapeutic for your varicocele. If you prepare properly, you can set up 8 hours of healing and greatly improve your treatment results! I place high emphasis on night-time treatment in my Personalized Treatment Plans. Do not overlook how effective this can be, not just for pain, but also for fertility and healing.

Sleeping Position

Every Night is Different: Feel your varicocele every night to see which position(s) or inversion(s) work best for you. Remember to relax and hold each position for 10 deep breaths and allow your body to adjust to the position before feeling your varicocele.

Quality Sleep

Here are some tips to improve your sleep quality: Take a warm shower before bed, drink a warm cup of milk, drink chamomile or other sleepy time teas, avoid caffeine, have a night-time snack, stretch, perform yoga, wear an eye mask, put in ear plugs, block out noise, make your sleeping environment comfortable, listen to soft music/music that you like, sleep with someone you trust in the room, see a sleep therapist, etc. The most important things are to sleep with someone that you trust, develop a set sleeping routine, find what works for you and stick to it, and have a set time to sleep every night and wake every morning.

Nighttime Inversion

Pillow Under Hips: It is very normal for the middle of the bed to sink in. This is not good for varicocele. So, what we can do is place a pillow under our hips to elevate them overnight. This greatly improves varicocele treatment results by both counteracting the negative effects of sunken in beds, and creating a small inversion that lasts many hours. This is a very effective treatment, do not underestimate it.

You can perform it by placing a medium sized pillow underneath your hips. You want your hips to be elevated about an inch higher than your torso. Fall asleep with the pillow underneath your hips, and simply remove it whenever you wake up to adjust at night. You do not have to force yourself to sleep with it all night. Perform 3-4 days a week. Stop this treatment if you experience neck or lower back discomfort.

Note: Do not have a pillow under your head if you place a place under your hips. This places excessive stress on your neck. Again, no pillow under your head when you have a pillow under your hips. You should also make to maintain length at the back of your neck by tucking your chin in slightly.

Bed Tilt: It is not good if the tilt of your bed holds your head higher than your legs (more upright is not good). This prevents nighttime inversion and is neither good for varicocele symptom treatment nor healing. It is more ideal if the tilt of your bed goes the other way; holding your legs higher than your head (more inverted is good). You do not want a big tilt, then a 1-2 degree tilt is good enough. The inversion should be barely noticeable.

Nocturnal Scrotal Cooling

Nocturnal Scrotal Cooling: Without proper cooling, sleep can become eight hours of testicular heat stress. We can to avoid as many testicular stressors as we can. Therefore, it is critical to ensure that normal testicular temperature is maintained during sleep.

Nocturnal cooling of only one degree Celsius (bellow the personal norm) is enough to improve sperm density, total sperm count, percentage of progressive motile spermatozoa and percentage of normally shaped spermatozoa after several weeks of treatment. What is shocking is that these results are better than surgical outcomes.

First, I recommend that you take time and perform an inversion for a few minutes to cool your varicocele fully before going to sleep. When sleeping, it is important to sleep bottomless or in thin/breathable pajama pants or underwear. Consider nocturnal scrotal cooling as the fundamental that you must practice daily.

Scrotal temperatures during lying on the sides or front are higher than lying on the back. Therefore, ideally, you want to sleep lying on your back. You cannot sleep on your back all night though. So, I recommend just wearing your circle-cut pants (read below) and not caring (as it will keep your testicles at a perfect temperature throughout the night). You can also sleep bottomless (without pants and underwear).

You can also consider using a cooling device or liquid cooling pack that you can purchase at a local pharmacy. As for the cooling pack, apply it for about 15 minutes in bed, before going to sleep. The cooling pack should not be too cold; it should just feel mildly cool to the touch. You may wrap the cooling pack in a towel if it is too cold. Apply the cooling pack at most five times per month.

Cool Your Room: These days our rooms are too warm. Lowering the temperature of your room is a great way reducing scrotal temperature both during the day and overnight.

Circle-Cut Pants:

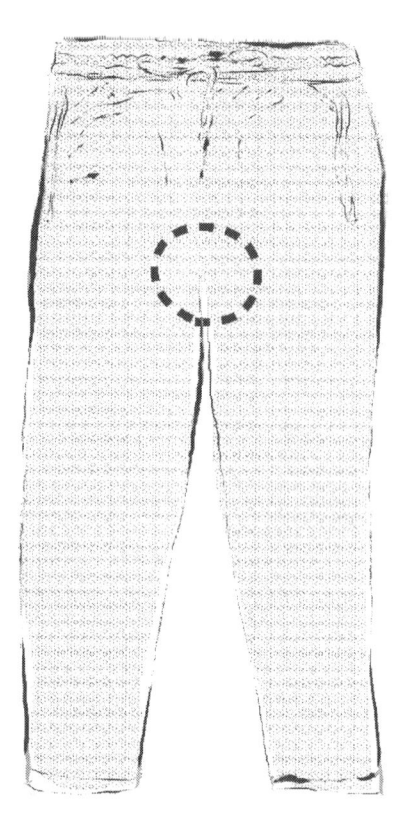

An easy way to ensure that your testicles are cool at night is to cut out a large circle out of the groin of your pants and use it when sleeping. The circle should be about 10 inches in diameter, ranging from just above your pubic bone to just before your anus. Make it big, but not too big. Your goal is to cool the general scrotal area.

Wearing circle Cut Pants is healthier and more effective than using a cooling pack. It is healthier because you do not have to worry about testicular hypothermia (overcooling your testicles); your testicles will self-regulate to their ideal temperature. It is more effective because you can use it every night, and all night. I highly recommend it for anyone who has varicocele pain or infertility. Think of it as fertility or therapeutic pants.

Thin & Breathable Pajamas: If you do not want to cut a circle out of your pants, it is also a good idea to invest in thin & breathable pajamas.

Note: Make sure that the waist is not tight at all, and if it is, cut it loose.

BE CAREFUL

Excessive Hot Tub, Sauna, Hot Showers, Etc.

There is nothing wrong with using a hot tub or sauna, and most definitely nothing wrong with hot showers. However, excessive or prolonged elevation of scrotal temperatures can have negative implications on pain and infertility. So, do your best to keep your testicles at a normal temperature on average, and reduce long-duration heating if it worsens your symptoms.

I should however make a note that early in your treatment (e.g. three to four weeks), it is ideal to minimize all stressors, and that means no hot tub or sauna. However, after the three to four weeks of treatment, once you have gained some good results, your testicles will be much healthier and more resilient to stress.

Testicular Hypothermia

Do not cause testicular hypothermia! You do not want to stress out your testicles! I cannot emphasize this enough. Your testicles are smaller than a golf-ball, and therefore their temperature can change very quickly. The best idea is to provide an optimal environment and allow them to regulate their own temperature.

Remember that your goal is to perform some cooling treatments and to on average normalize testicular temperature—not cause testicular hypothermia!

Cold & Warm Water Alternations

Cold and warm water alternations can help reduce varicocele pain and swelling and help improve vein contractility. They should however be performed with caution as they can worsen your symptoms if done incorrectly.

Simply alternate between running cold and warm water over your testicles & varicocele. Each alternation should take about 5-10 seconds.

Caution: Make sure to always end this treatment with the cold alternation. Also, use water that is not is just warm (not hot) for the warm water alternation.

Non-Steroidal Anti-Inflammatory Drugs
Ibuprofen/Advil is often prescribed to help attain temporary relief from varicocele pain. If your symptoms are severe, you should consult your physician about the appropriateness of taking it.

The one note that I will make is that Ibuprofen/Advil and similar products are known to cause stomach and digestive problems, and other negative side-effects that may actually be worsen your varicocele symptoms. These products should be taken with caution and attention to side-effects.

OTHER

Cognitive Behavioral Therapy (CBT)
I was surprised recently when I found out that CBT is just as effective as surgery at reducing varicocele pain. If you do receive CBT, do not use it as a substitute for the other treatments in this guide; make sure perform both CBT and the other treatments recommended in this guide.

Cool Down Your Environment
If you can, it is ideal to cool down your room or work environment by 1-2°C/2-4°F. This makes it much easier to manage your testicular temperature.

MAYBE SOMETHING ELSE IS CAUSING YOUR SYMPTOMS
If you have not seen your physician to rule out any other causes for your symptoms other than varicocele, then you need to do so. You should also note that the following symptoms may indicate a different a condition than varicocele: Pain when urinating, pain in the penis shaft, pain in the lower abdomen or lower back, sharp and shooting pain, pain that is increasing and not deceasing, sudden onset of pain, increase of pain with treatments,

swelling of the scrotum and not veins, testicular swelling, etc. If you experience any of the above symptoms, or any symptoms that seem odd, see your physician or a specialist.

Chronic Mild Epididymitis

Chronic mild epididymitis is an underdiagnosed and sometimes difficult to detect condition that may be either the cause of your varicocele swelling or scrotal pain. If you think that you have this condition, you should see your physician before continuing.

Aside from medical treatment, you can use the following strategies to minimize your risk of developing epididymitis and reduce the severity of its symptoms: Use safe sex practices, have good hygiene, and perform anti-inflammatory treatments.

Safe sex practices: Have sex with only one partner at a time, make sure that your partner is tested and uninfected, use a condom every time, and do not share any sex toys.

Good Hygiene: Wash your penis properly and regularly (especially if you have foreskin), urinate and wash your penis and testicles after sex, and drink plenty of water and fluids daily.

Anti-inflammatory Treatments: Perform a cooling treatment or inversion to reduce swelling and pain.

CHAPTER DEFINITIONS

Cremaster Muscle: The muscle of that wraps around the testicles.

Cremaster Reflex: The cremaster muscle contracts and pulls the testicles up when cold, exercising, or erect.

Epididymis: A lump on your testicles that supports sperm development.

Epididymitis: Swelling of the epididymis.

Genital Heat Stress: Stress and damage caused by elevated scrotal/testicular temperature.

Hyperthermia: Too much heat, or over-heating.

Hypothermia: Too little heat, or over-cooling.

Intra-Abdominal Pressure: The pressure that is inside your torso. You want to minimize and manage this pressure.

Normal Testicular Temperature: Testicular temperature when adequate heat exchange and circulation are allowed (34-36°C/93.5-96.5°F).

DANIEL JOHNSON

CHAPTER 3

LIFESTYLE CHANGES

In treating your varicocele, you will have to make some lifestyle changes. These changes are simple, but they can have a profound impact on the status of your varicocele and the treatment process. It is very important to take a holistic approach to varicocele treatment. Do not overly focus on varicocele-specific treatments. Make the important lifestyle changes outlined in this chapter, and you will get major benefits for your varicocele.

STOP CIGARETTES, ALCOHOL & COFFEE

Cigarettes

Over and over again, studies show that cigarette smoking reduces sperm count, density, and motility, and leads to higher abnormalities in sperm shape and function. It also relates to higher rates of hormonal issues and erectile dysfunction.

Relative to varicocele, cigarette smoking may increase varicocele pain, is known to have a large negative impact on fertility, leads to hormone dysfunctions, and testicular shrinkage. Cigarettes increase blood toxicity and make blood stickier (less able to flow smoothly). Since varicocele impedes testicular blood circulation, it is important to optimize blood circulation and quality; not to impair it.

There is good news: Studies have found improvements of all fertility and hormone parameters in those who stop cigarette smoking.

Alcohol

Alcohol is a leading cause of erectile dysfunction. It lowers testosterone levels, libido, and negatively affects many of the same parameters as smoking. Related to the varicocele, alcohol overloads the liver (which is responsible for filtering blood), makes your blood more viscous (thick), and increases the cardiac output (causing the heart to pump more blood). Pumping more and thicker blood will increase the amount of blood that will pool in your varicocele.

Coffee

Relative to your varicocele, coffee (or caffeine) may be worsening your symptoms. Caffeine causes a mildly anxious state that lasts for hours (until the caffeine filters out of your system). The half-life for caffeine in your body is six hours. This means if you drink a cup of coffee with 140 mg of caffeine at 10 AM, by 4 PM your body still has 70 mg of caffeine. By 10 PM you still have 35 mg of caffeine in your system. Meaning that by the time you go to bed at 10 PM, you still have the equivalent of a quarter of a cup of coffee in your body.

The mildly anxious state lasts almost as long as you have caffeine in your system. Caffeine is a drug that acts directly on the brain by stimulating the sympathetic pathway (fight or flight response). The sympathetic pathway is bad for digestion, sleep, and healing! Now, consider that caffeine causes thinning of the stomach mucous lining, irritable bowel syndrome, insomnia, and is related to lymphatic swelling.

I especially recommend staying away from coffee if you are a smoker or heavy alcohol drinker because evidence suggests that comorbidity is higher in mixed users.

It is up to you to make the changes necessary for improving your health.

HEALTHY MASTURBATION
Healthy Masturbation (Dos):

+ Lay down while masturbating
+ Lay down 10-20 minutes after masturbating
+ Sleep after masturbating/masturbate at night before sleep
+ Allow adequate post-masturbation cooling
+ Have some days/periods without masturbation
+ Play with & stimulate your testicles
+ For optimal fertility, ejaculate once every 2-3 days
+ Avoid physically rubbing or tugging your testicular veins
+ Sex is okay
+ Ideally, perform a cooling treatment after masturbation and sex

Unhealthy Masturbation (Do Not Dos):
+ Masturbate while sitting and/or sit after masturbation (e.g. when watching porn)
+ Squeeze your penis aggressively and tightly
+ Masturbate before exercise, strenuous activity, going out, or travel
+ Masturbate more than three times per day OR masturbate multiple times, every single day
+ Perform penis enlargement exercises without caution
+ Take Viagra

NO & Masturbation: Recent research has shown that excess Nitric Oxide (NO) is released from the testicular veins. Excess NO is toxic, impairs fertility, increases vein diameter, is associated with higher grade varicocele, and varicocele progression with age.

Excess masturbation may lead to excess NO production in surrounding tissue. Even after masturbating once, varicose veins typically swell, the testicles heat up and the cremaster muscle relaxes. Pooling of blood, in this case, is not the cause of faulty valves but of excessive NO production, elevated temperature, and a low hanging scrotum, all in combination with increased blood flow to the testicles.

Ejaculation Frequency & Fertility: Not ejaculating at all leads to increased concentration of old sperm which are damaged by toxic and oxidizing agents. It takes sixty days for your sperm to mature. Ejaculation gets rid of old damaged sperm and improves the concentration of new, healthy, and mature sperm. For optimal fertility, you should ejaculate once every 2-3 days. Do not ejaculate too frequently as this depletes sperm count.

Avoid Aggressive Tugging: Tugging on your skin while masturbating (especially if you are circumcised), can also tug on your varicose testicular veins. This can irritate them and make them more sensitive to pain. Instead, masturbate softly and use lubrication. In addition, excessive and aggressive masturbation (especially without lubrication) irritates the skin and glans, and reduces glans sensitivity. Reduced sensitivity leads to easily lost erections, less enjoyment of sex, and a condition you might have heard about from a bragging friend, where he lasts hours without being able to climax.

Do Not Use a Tight Grip: Squeezing your hand tightly around your shaft when you masturbate (masturbating with a tight grip) causes excess pressure that can irritate your varicocele and make it more prone to aching. It is okay to use a tighter grip if you are lying down or are in an inversion.

Stop PE Exercises: Stop all natural penis enlargement (PE) exercises, as they often contribute to varicocele development and symptom severity. If you do choose to continue PE exercises, do so with caution. Remember to minimize excessive pressure, keep your testicles cool, and do not tug on or rub the veins aggressively.

CONSTIPATION & BOWELS

Interestingly, there is a difference in the occurrence of varicosities (including varicocele) in developed countries versus developing countries. Developing countries have much lower rates of varicosities. This discrepancy is largely due to the difference in diet and lifestyle.

Chronic Constipation

Chronic constipation is one of the most common functional gastrointestinal disorders, affecting up to 27% of the North American population. Chronic constipation can cause varicocele to develop.

Pushing hard to have a bowel movement increases intra-abdominal venous pressure. Moreover, constipation typically comes with irregular bowel movements. This literally means that there is a build-up of feces in the intestines (exacerbating the nutcracker effect). In the long-term, these risk factors contribute to both varicocele development and severity.

For optimal bowel movements, you have to manage your stress, diet, hydration, activity, and maybe consider a few supplements.

Stress: Stress can cause many negative bodily symptoms, including irregular bowel movements, constipation, inflammatory bowel syndrome, and irritable bowel syndrome. It is a major factor you have to get under control, see Chapter 4: Fertility & Sexual Health for more details.

Diet: You really have to look at your stool in the toilet. If it is too hard, maybe you need more indigestible fiber from vegetables. If it is not smooth enough, you might need more volume from legumes (e.g. beans, lentils, chickpeas, etc.). If it falls apart too easily, maybe you need more sticky food like oats and oily food in your diet, and less acidic and hard to digest food. If your food does not digest well, maybe you should have more yogurt, or other fermented food with probiotics.

Hydration: Dehydration is also a major cause of dry, hard stools. As food passes through your intestines, the moisture from it is soaked up. This is even more pronounced when you are dehydrated since your body wants to retain as much water as possible.

Activity: You need to move to stimulate bowel movement. Exercising, in general, especially inversions, twist and some of the ones recommended later in this guide are very helpful. Even going out for a walk can be very stimulating for a bowel movement.

Supplements: Consider taking a vitamin D supplement if you do not get at least 15 minutes of direct sunlight daily, as it is important for proper digestion and reducing bowel inflammation. You could also try digestive enzymes and probiotic supplements (you might have to experiment with different probiotic cultures to see which works best with your digestive system).

Stool softeners can help alleviate constipation and may even be necessary early on for addressing chronic constipation. Keep in mind that you have to drink a lot of water if you take stool softeners, and that they should not serve substitute for a fiber-rich and healthy diet.

Bloated Digestive System
Digestive health is not only vitally important only for your varicocele but also for your overall health.

Bloating is a very common digestive disease. The main cause of bloating is stress. Other major contributors to bloating include lack of exercise, poor diet, and eating on the go. Activity and exercise are important bowel health (will be discussed in more detail). A diet low in probiotics, and high in processed food and sugar tends to cause bloating. Eating too quickly, then exercising or running the day's tasks can irritate the digestive system, leading to bloating.

Probiotics
Did you know that the human body contains 10 times more bacterial cells than human cells? So, from that, it is not hard to understand why upsetting the bacterial balance can cause many disorders. Our focus is on digestion, and probiotics are vitally important to that. You need to have some fermented food as a regular part of your diet. I am not talking about artificially sweetened yogurt, what I mean is fermented food like miso, natto, tempeh, kimchi, pickled food, sauerkraut, chutneys, and low fat plain white yogurt.

Lymph
Disturbances in the lymphatic system may also contribute to or be the cause of some cases of varicocele. Specifically, we are concerned with the enlargement of the groin lymph nodes (in the retroperitoneum space) and inadequate lymph drainage. Enlargement of these lymph nodes impedes spermatic vein blood flow and causes the development of varicocele. Improper lymph drainage also leads to immune system and digestive problems.

The lymphatic system is an intricate system much like the venous system. It branches and reaches almost the entire body. Its major functions are cleaning out waste products and fighting invading bacteria or viruses. Therefore, swelling of the lymph typically is indicative of high levels of toxicity or foreign invaders.

Unlike the venous system, the lymphatic system is not pumped throughout the body by a pump like the heart. Instead, it relies mainly on the flexion and relaxation of surrounding muscular tissue to flow. Therefore, it is important to breathe deeply through your stomach and to have a physically active lifestyle.

More specific to varicocele, you want to perform your abdominal exercises and stimulate and strengthen the lower abs (covered in more detail in Chapter 6: Fitness & Exercises).

COUGHING

It is good to be aware that coughing increases intra-abdominal venous pressure and can therefore irritate your varicocele and worsen your symptoms.

Since the causes of chronic cough vary greatly, I recommend consulting a qualified physician for more information.

Some cough you can control. For example, if you live in a city that has particularly dry air that irritates your airway, you can purchase a humidifier for your home, moisturize your nostrils saltwater or cream.

SQUATTING ON THE TOILET

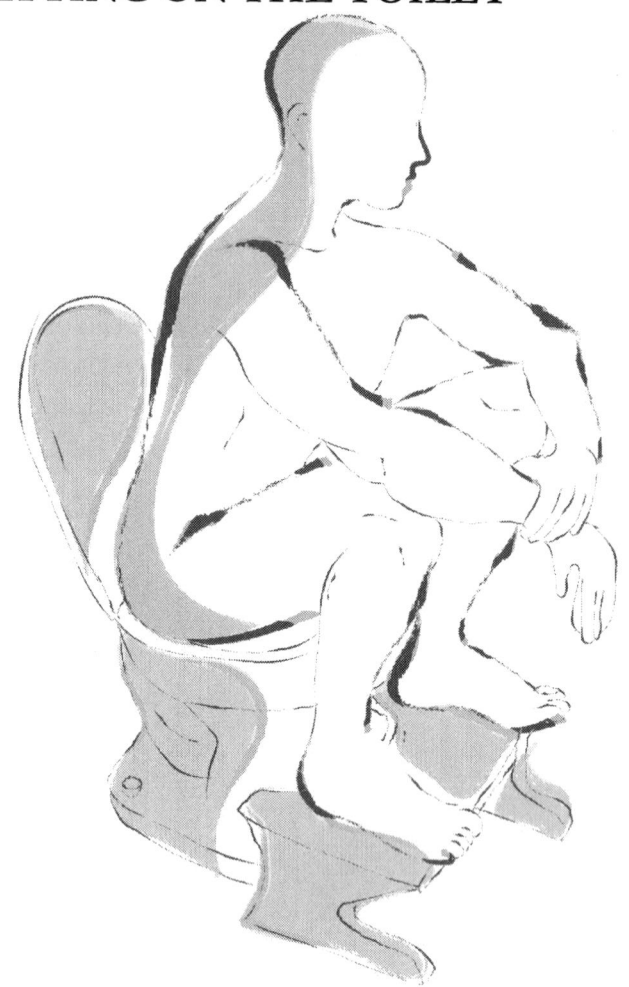

Toilets are unnatural for bowel movement. They force a posture that pinches and hinders the natural flow of stools. This means excess pressure as you push and force the stool out and only partial emptying of the bowels. This is a very important and easy change to make. Correcting this is equivalent to for controlling one of the stress factors that contribute to varicocele development. Squatting on the toilet is very healthy, you will also instantly notice the difference in the ease of your bowel movements! I cannot emphasize how big of a difference a few simple lifestyle changes can make.

The idea is to raise your knees up and tilt your torso forward so that your body is in more of a squatting position. Similar to the position used for Eastern squatting toilets. To raise your knees up into a squatter position, you could buy a squatting stool, but I recommend buying yoga foam blocks instead because they are less strange to keep around the washroom. However, you can really use anything to prop up your legs.

If you do not have access to anything to prop up your legs, bend over closer to your knees; do not sit up straight.

To further enhance ease with which the stool flows, bend over your legs slightly (do not sit up straight), spread your butt cheeks (grab and roll them out), and relax.

CHAPTER DEFINITIONS

Bowel Movement: The act of defecating.

Bowels: All of the digestive organs in the abdominal region.

Lymph: A clear-to-white fluid that forms in bodily tissue.

Lymphatic System: A network of vessels that have functions for the immune system and fluid retention.

Penis Enlargement (PE) Exercises: Any exercise, stretch, or treatment that is aimed to enlarge the penis or testicles.

Probiotic: Any microorganism that has beneficial qualities for the body.

DANIEL JOHNSON

CHAPTER 4

FERTILITY & SEXUAL HEALTH

CHAPTER INTRO

More than one in four people with varicocele experience fertility problems. That is about 2-4% of the population! The main parameters used for assessing fertility are sperm count, volume, morphology, and motility, as well as sperm DNA damage and testicular volume. Varicocele can negatively affect all these parameters.

Varicocele can also cause a decrease in testosterone levels, leading to decreased sexual performance, and slight feminization of the body and mind (e.g. enlargement of breast tissue, erectile dysfunction, passivity, and decreased assertiveness).

To improve fertility, you must relieve testicular hyperthermia, improve testicular blood flow (to reduce reactive oxygen species, and remove toxins), improve your diet, and normalize your hormones. Fertility and hormones are very closely connected. For example, the testicles need to be healthy to stimulate testosterone release, while testosterone release is required for testicular health, and sperm development.

Testicular volume is a strong predictor of both fertility and normal hormone balance. Lower testicular volume is common in those diagnosed with a varicocele. Normal volume is normally greater than 15 cm^3. Varicocele causes an average decrease of 5 cm^3 of volume on the affected side. Notably the unaffected side may also shrink because of disruptions in hormone balance on the effected side. Higher grade or bilateral varicoceles cause the greatest decrease in testicular volume.

Your testicles have a particular firmness to them when they are healthy. Notice that they have a nice healthy feel when you take care of them and in contrast, a soggy and droopy feel when stressed. As you follow this guide, you will notice that the affected side's firmness will return.

This section has exercises specifically select for improving fertility and stimulating testicular growth. However, do not neglect the other chapters of the book; they contain varicocele specific treatments and will therefore also contribute to your recovery and results.

ALLEVIATE VARICOCELE INDUCED DAMAGE & STRESS

Cool

Sperm density decreases by 40% for each degree Celsius increase of average daily scrotal temperatures. In fact, testicle temperatures above 36.5°C/98°F completely halt sperm production.

Varicocele damages the counter current heat exchange mechanism of the pampiniform plexus. This means chronically elevated testicular temperature, leading to damaged testicles and impaired fertility.

To improve your fertility, you should aim to both normalized your testicular temperature, and perform some cooling treatments (see Chapter 2: Cooling & Pain Relief for more details).

Circulate

Pooled blood is toxic to the testicles and impairs fertility for many reasons. Varicocele pools blood in the testicular veins. Therefore, to improve fertility, you must perform inversions regularly (see Chapter 2: Cooling & Pain Relief for more details).

Antioxidants

Reactive oxygen species (ROS) damage sperm and sperm DNA. Varicocele impairs nutrient exchange, and toxin removal from the testicles, elevates testicular temperature, and increases ROS concentration in the testicles. All of these lead to increased ROS activity and therefore damage fertility.

There is a lot of scientific evidence stating that a diet high in antioxidants or antioxidant supplementation can help improve fertility and reduce sperm DNA damage in those with varicocele. Therefore, if you want to improve your fertility, you must make sure to increase the amount of antioxidants in your diet (see Chapter 5: Diet & Nutrition for more details).

IMPROVE TESTICULAR HEALTH

Testicle Massage

Testicle Massage is a great treatment for increasing blood flow to your testicles to stimulating their growth, improve fertility, and boost testosterone. This treatment may aggravate your condition if your varicocele is inflamed or you have testicular pain However, when practiced properly, it is great for improving fertility, returning firmness to your testicles, and restoring lost testicular size. Also, in the long-term, it can help reduce pain originating from the testicles.

Testicular size and firmness are clear indicators of how healthy your testicles are. It is easy to know when your testicles healthy. When you lightly squeeze them, you can tell that they have a nice, firm, and plump feel to them. The same is true about the scrotum; when it is healthy, it has a nice healthy texture, rather than a saggy and droopy one.

Only perform this treatment while lying on your back with your legs on the wall. Doing so will drain your varicose veins and protect them from the light tugging and rubbing that is caused by the treatment. I recommend that you perform this treatment at night, and only after a minimum of 5 minute inversion (pre-treatment).

To begin this treatment, grab one of your testicles in one hand, and lightly moving it away from your body. Only move it as far away as you need to perform the treatment. This is the starting position. Now, using both palms, massage your testicle by rolling it as if you are making a ball out of Playdough (or dough). Massage gently. Keep rolling your testicle gently for about 2 minutes. Then perform the same treatment on the other testicle. Perform this treatment 1-2 times a week.

Important Notes: Do not perform this treatment when in pain or when your varicocele is swollen. Only perform it in an inversion (e.g. feet up on the wall). Perform gently. Ideally, perform both a minimum 5 minute inversion post-treatment, and some sort of cooling treatment after that massage.

Oil Massage

An oil massage can be very nurturing for the testicles and can help reduce varicocele inflammation. I recommend using olive oil, coconut oil, or hemp seed oil because of their nurturing and anti-inflammatory properties. This treatment is the same as the Testicle Massage (the previous treatment), however is done with the application of oil.

An added benefit to this treatment is that it can help improve scrotal skin tone, has anti-inflammatory benefits for the skin, alleviates stress from the area, and stimulates healthy blood flow to the testicles and surrounding tissue. These are all great for fertility and long-term healing.

Begin by applying the oil to your hands and gently massage your testicles. You can also rub the oil in and around the scrotal skin (including over the varicocele). Continue for 2-3 minutes. Perform 1-2 times a week.

Important Notes: Do not perform this treatment when in pain or when your varicocele is swollen. Only perform it in an inversion (e.g. feet up on the wall). Perform gently. Ideally, perform both a minimum 5 minute inversion post-treatment, and some sort of cooling treatment after that massage.

Boost Testosterone

Low testosterone can lead to testicular atrophy, low semen volume, erectile dysfunction, and decreased libido. For healthy testicles, you must normalize or boost testosterone levels. Some proven methods of naturally boosting testosterone include dietary changes (see Chapter 5: Diet & Nutrition) physical activity, lower body fat, having sex frequently, sleeping well, and better stress management.

Quality Sleep
Sleeping well at night is critically important maintaining and improving testicular health. Poor sleep is linked to both infertility and testicular atrophy. Relevant also to fertility and varicocele, you must make sure to keep your testicles at a normal temperature throughout the night, and make sure that your bed supports healthy blood circulation. Please refer to Chapter 2: Cooling & Pain Relief for more details.

Stress Management
The more stressed you are the less blood, energy, and nutrients are dedicated to your sexual and digestive organs, and immune system. This means poor testicular health and impaired fertility. Therefore, it is critical to manage your stress. Stress management is discussed further later in this chapter.

Keep Active
Regular physical activity is critically important for keeping your testicles healthy. It helps improve testicular blood flow, boost testosterone, and stimulate fertility. So, find more reasons to be active. Exercise in the mornings, walk regularly, join a sports, dance, or activity club, and make friend and family gatherings more active than sedentary. See Chapter 6: Fitness & Exercises for more details.

Normal Weight
Overweight and obesity have a large negative impact on testicular health because they increase testicular temperature, lower testosterone, increase testicular pressure, decrease nutrition, and increase toxicity. See Chapter 4: Fitness & Exercises and Chapter 5: Diet & Nutrition for more details.

Healing & Meditative Practices
Healing and meditative practices increase healthy blood flow to the testicles, help alleviate stress, and place the body in a healing state. I recommend yoga, acupuncture, tai chi, qi gong, therapeutic massage, Chinese herbal medicine, mind-body practices, etc. These practices reduce genital inflammatory conditions, improve sperm parameters, modulate the immune system, and improve sexual and ejaculatory function.

An interesting side note is that many scientific studies have found that the above healing & meditative practices are just as effective as surgery in improving fertility, but carry none of the associated risks as surgery and have many other positive benefits.

SEXUAL HEALTH

Penile Health

These exercises are great for improving erections, sexual performance, and overall penis health. They also help maintain and strengthen the ligaments and tendons of the pelvic floor by relieving excess tension, and pressure built by knots and stiffness in the tissue.

Kegels: One of the most well-recognized exercises for naturally enhancing penile health and performance, is the kegel (also known as the pelvic floor exercise). Over the past 60 years, it has been repeatedly demonstrated to be effective at improving fertility and erections and enhancing sexual performance. It is also beneficial for the prostate gland, testicles, pelvic floor muscle, and may be effective for reducing varicocele-related pain.

To perform a kegel, tense the same muscles you use when you stop urinating. These are the muscles of the pelvic floor, including the pubococcygeus muscle (commonly referred to as the PC muscle). Perform either 10 repetitions of 10-second holds, with brief rests, or 100 repetitions of one-second holds (both are effective). I recommend performing this exercise three to five times a week for two months, then winding down to once a week.

Those without varicocele can perform this exercise anywhere. However, I recommend that those with varicocele perform this exercise while lying down or with legs up on the wall (in an inversion). An inversion will help alleviate the excess pressure that this exercise produces in the lower abdomen and pelvic region.

Note that some people have a sensitive or overactive pelvic floor muscle and should not perform kegel exercises without the aid of a qualified physiotherapist.

Flaccid Penis Stretch: The flaccid (soft) penis stretch help lengthen the penis and improve erections. In addition, it helps increase libido and testosterone to a small degree.

For this this stretch, begin lying on your back, with your legs spread slightly, and knees bent. Start by grabbing your penis on the upper part of the shaft, close to the penis head. Now, pull your penis until you feel a medium intensity stretch. Pull your penis up, down, left, right, and straight out. Hold each direction for 5 to 10 seconds. Once done, Switch hands and repeat the sequence one more time. You can perform this stretch as often as you like. It is especially effective after long hours of sitting, standing, running or biking.

Erect Penis Stretch: Stretching your penis when it is erect (hard) has very similar benefits to the flaccid penis stretch, however it also helps improve penis girth (thickness) and is more suited for erection hardness.

Perform the same way as the flaccid penis stretch, however, perform with 50-70% of full erection.

Cautionary note: Make sure that that you perform this stretch while in an inversion to minimize irritation of your varicocele.

Perineum Massage & Self-Acupressure: The perineum refers to the area below the abdomen and between the thighs and anus. Stretching and massaging the perineum improves blood circulation to the entire genitals, relieves tension (by alleviating tension from and improving circulation in the hips and legs), and enhances testosterone release, sex drive, and is beneficial for erections.

This treatment is especially effective after long hours of sitting, standing, running, or biking.

Down the center of the perineum, you will feel a rope or rod-like structure. This is the continuation of your penis. While lying down, gently massage either side of this rod. Massage with several fingers at once, slightly digging your fingers around and under the rod. Be careful to not massage your varicose veins, because doing so might irritate them.

This treatment should take about one to two minutes, and be performed only once per week.

Note: Do not press too hard or aggressively when performing this treatment.

Clean Urethra: Bacterial, viral, and fungal infections can severely inflame your varicose veins. For some, much of their varicocele pain and swelling, as well as sexual dysfunctions are due to chronic mild epididymitis, prostatitis, urinary tract infections, or recurrent heavy infections.

Drinking a lot of water is a great way to keep the urinary tract clean. It increases urine volume, and frequency, flushing out any foreign invaders, and keeping the urinary tract clean.

You should also be taking preventative measure to keep your urethra clear of foreign invaders, for example, always use a condom during sexual activity, only have one sex partner, get tested for sexually transmitted infections regularly, minimize risky sexual activity, do not share any sex toys, etc.

Cardiovascular Health: Poor cardiovascular health is a major cause of erectile dysfunctions, and contributes to poor overall sexual health. See Chapter 6: Fitness & Exercises for more details.

Diet & Nutrition: Diet and nutrition play a big role in virility. When it comes to virility, there are many effective herbs, supplements, roots, etc. that you can take.

Prostate Health

The prostate gland is located deep of the perineum and is responsible for producing prostatic fluid, which is the part of the ejaculate that helps semen motility. Good prostate health is critical for fertility.

Not So Regular Ejaculations: According to science ejaculating once every two to three days is ideal for fertility, and five to seven times a week is ideal for long-term prostate health. However, I believe that a lower number is ideal for those with varicocele.

Lower frequency of masturbation, especially early on in your treatment, will help reduce excessive blood flow to the testicles. This means less blood pooling. Less blood pooling means less toxic damage, testosterone reflux, and better nutrient exchange for the testicles and prostate. In my opinion, this will do much more for your prostate health than regular ejaculations.

Prostate Self-Acupressure: This is a gentle self-acupressure to stimulate the prostate gland. This treatment helps improve erections and ejaculate volume.

To stimulate the prostate, follow the rod down to the area just before your anus. If you poke into this area, you should feel a soft section, roughly the size of the tip of your finger. Gently poke into and massage this area. Perform this exercise for 30 seconds, maximum once a week.

Note: Discontinue this treatment if you develop any discomfort.

Kegels: As mentioned earlier, kegels are great for overall sexual health. Kegeling also increases blood flow to the prostate gland and helps improve prostate health. To perform a kegel, follow the guidelines earlier in this chapter.

Healthy Weight & Regular Activity: Physical activity is associated with prostate health. While you can benefit from any form of physical activity (even walking), cardiovascular activity has the highest benefits for prostate health.

Diet & Prostate: I will be adding some information on this in the next edition of the Healing Guide.

PREGNANCY TIPS

When it comes to fertility and pregnancy, you really have too many treatment options! Do not get stuck in the surgery vs embolization marketing gimmick! In the next edition of the Healing Guide, I will write 100+ fertility and pregnancy tips for you. I want you to know that you have options!

STRESS MANAGEMENT

Stress can have a huge negative global impact on the body. Relevant to varicocele, it can impair healthy blood flow, reduce the effectiveness of digestion and bowel movements, and has a direct negative impact on fertility.

Stress impairs healthy blood flow because it reduces the amount of nutrients in the blood, increases blood acidity, may cause high blood pressure, and decreases blood flow to digestive and reproductive organs. All of these create a dysfunctional environment that stagnates healing and hinders optimal testicular function.

Stress increases inflammation and bloating, suppresses normal digestion, reduces the number of bowel movements (suppresses the urge to defecate), increases bowel irregularly, and is associated with irritable bowel syndrome. All this is bad because it leads to irregular and less frequent bowel movements, inflammation of the gut, and higher pressure in the midsection. Therefore, stress can have a significant contribution to varicocele development and severity.

Stress can also directly decrease fertility because it reduces testosterone production. Testosterone is required for normal spermatogenesis (sperm development). Moderate to severe stress is associated with a 40-50% decrease in sperm count, and a lowering of the total number of motile sperm.

If you follow the rest of this guide but you do not manage your stress, you will greatly reduce the effectiveness of all the treatments. So, you must manage your stress.

Proper stress management is a skill. It is preventative, preparative, and regulatory. You must take action in order to prevent outcomes that will cause you stress, prepare and have readiness for outcomes that you cannot control, and regulate stress when it arises. Again, proper stress management is a skill. That means it requires education, and long-term practice to improve.

HEALTHY WEIGHT

Surprisingly, as body mass index (BMI) increases, varicocele grade and severity decreases. That means that overweight and obese individuals have lower incidence of varicocele and less severe symptoms. It is thought that this is the case because abdominal fat helps cushion and lesson the severity of the nutcracker effect.

I obviously do not recommend becoming overweight or obese for varicocele treatment or improvement in fertility.

When compared to those with normal weight, obese men on average are 42% more likely to have low sperm count, have on average 24% lower sperm count, and are 81% more likely to be sterile. Moreover, for every three-point increase in BMI, above normal weight, male infertility decreases by about 10%. Being obese also comes with a many other problems that negatively affect overall health.

To me, the health risks associated with being overweight and obese far outweigh the positive effect it may have on varicocele. Therefore, I recommend that you eat healthy and exercise frequently to attain and maintain a healthy weight.

Two advice is almost always given for weight management. First you must eat healthy, and second you must exercise frequently.

To eat healthy, cut out the fast food, junk food, sugary food and drinks, and overly processed food. Make your diet balanced and wholesome. Research what food is good for you, and what food is bad for you. Always have some healthy food that you enjoy handy. You would be surprised at how quickly your weight changes once you make dietary changes.

Here are some tips to exercise more frequently: If you do not have a gym membership, get one. Go to the gym at least three to four days a week, consistently, for at least three months to notice results. You do not have to work out like crazy. The most important thing is just being consistent with going to the gym. Consistency is key. It is very helpful to join a regular, scheduled, group activity. Later, you can gradually begin to research what exercises are most effective and how best to perform them. Take it easy and just be consistent.

Follow this simple advice (eat health and exercise consistently) and you will attain a healthy weight with relative ease.

CHAPTER DEFINITIONS

Body Mass Index (BMI): A simple method of categorizing people's weight relative to their height. The formula is weight in kilograms divided by height in meters squared.

Defecate: Discharge feces from the body.

Flaccid: When the penis is soft and limp.

Girth: The circumference or thickness of the penis.

Perineum: The region from the pubic bone and anus that is between the legs.

Self-Acupressure: Pressing into specific areas with your fingers to stimulate blood flow and therapeutic effects.

Stress: Anything that resists your being exerts stress on your system.

Testicular Shrinkage/Atrophy: A condition where the testicle reduces in size.

Urethra: The duct through which you urinate.

DANIEL JOHNSON

CHAPTER 5

DIET & NUTRITION

VARICOCELE HEALING

A good diet with proper nutrition will make a big difference in healing and reducing negative symptoms. Relevant to healing and optimizing fertility, a good diet consists of food that improves circulatory and venous health, is anti-inflammatory, high in antioxidants, optimizes testosterone production, and aids in digestion.

I recommend trying out a few different supplements. The supplements I recommend are inexpensive, have little or no side effects, and have scientifically proven efficacy. I highly recommend at least testing them out. Many of the recommended supplements are anti-inflammatory, help strengthen connective tissue that support veins, contain vascular tonifying agents, and have chemicals that help develop, and support good vascular and circulatory health.

Note that I have not recommended any doses for the recommended supplements. From my experience, doses recommended by most companies are not very different from the doses used in research. Try at least a few of these supplements, but do not take too many at once.

Caution: These supplements may interact with certain medications. They may cause negative side effects and worsen some conditions. Make sure to consult a qualified healthcare practitioner before starting any supplement.

Healing Supplements

Horse Chestnut: Horse chestnut seed extract (active ingredient aescin) is very effective at treating varicosities. It has vasculoprotective properties, is anti-inflammatory, and a strong antioxidant. It is great for strengthening venous connective tissue, and vein walls. As well, it helps tighten the tissue surrounding the veins, helping increase vascular tone.

Bioflavonoids (Grape Seed and Pine Bark): Bioflavonoid supplementation is effective for treatment of venous insufficiency (varicosities). Bioflavonoids are vasculoprotective (because of their antioxidant properties), reduce inflammation and pain, improve venous tone and elasticity, protect connective tissue structure, increase vascular permeability and function, and improve capillary strength and effectiveness. Furthermore, some evidence suggests that bioflavonoids slow the progression of varicocele from subclinical to palpable.

The most effective bioflavonoids are diosmin, oligomeric proanthocyanidin complexes, and hesperidin. Grape seed and pine bark extract are high all of these bioflavonoids.

Butcher's Broom: Butcher's Broom has a long history of use in folk medicine for treatment of inflammation and varicosities. Now, scientific evidence also backs its efficacy. Butcher's broom maintains venous tone, enhances venous emptying, and improves blood circulation. It also is effective for treating constipation and abnormal water retention. Overall, Butcher's broom is effective for improving blood circulation and increasing blood vessel tightness and strength.

Gotu Kola: Gotu Kola is a plant supplement with a fair amount of scientific backing for its effectiveness at treating varicosities. It greatly enhances connective tissue integrity, elevates antioxidant levels in wound healing, and is generally good for vascular integrity.

Witch Hazel: Some evidence suggests that Witch Hazel may be beneficial for varicocele because it is anti-inflammatory, has antioxidant properties, and may help increase the contractility of veins.

Anti-Inflammatory Diet
Anti-inflammatory food help reduce excessive varicocele swelling and stimulate healing of varicose veins. Your diet should consist of food high in

anti-inflamatories, such as beats, berries, cellery, cabbage, cooked tomatoes, garlic, onions, ginger, kale, olive oil, flax seed oil, cod liver oil, nuts (especially walnuts and brazil nuts), whole grians, buckwheat, fatty fish, whole grains, dark leafy greens, chili, cayanne, tumeric, green tea, astax, aloe, mushrooms, etc.

Note that probiotics can help reduce gut inflamation. You should experiment with different probiotics to see which works best for you.

Avoid Inflammatory Food

You should be minimizing the amount of inlammatory food that you eat, and aware of any food sensativity or allergy (e.g. to milk, dairy products, gluten, animal proteins and fat, peanuts, etc.) that you may have. Inflamatroy foods include high fat dairy, alcohol, sugar, saturated and trans fats (e.g. sunflower, corn, and vegetable oils, margarine, etc.), imblanace of omega-6 and omega-3 fatty acids (high oemga-6 combined with low omega-3), refined carbohydrates (e.g. white flour products, white rice, pasta, etc.), artificial food coloring, MSG (monosodium glutamate), etc.

Diet Rich in Bioflavonoids

As mentioned earlier, bioflavonoids have many benefits for varicocele treatment. Food high in bioflavonoids include oranges, apples, apricots, blueberries, bilberries, cranberries, black currants, raspberries, strawberries, cherries, tomatoes, pears, parsley, tomatoes, onions, peppers, buckwheat, tea (green and black), and vegetables (white, yellow and orange). Your diet should contain food high in bioflavonoids.

BOWEL & DIGESTIVE HEALTH

Ideally, you want soft, well-formed, and regular bowel movements. The idea is to minimize the fullness of your bowels, and time spent in forceful Valsalva maneuver (holding breath and exerting). A well-formed stool is one that literally slides out of the anus. Anything else is really constipation.

When following this section on improving bowel movements, please remember that it is important to have a healthy and balanced diet. If you have further questions or concerns, consult a qualified healthcare practitioner.

Stool Volume

Increasing stool volume is important for smoothing and moistening bowels, may also normalize stickiness of stools, and is crucial for making bowel movements more regular and timelier (normalizes transit time of bowel movements).

To increase stool volume, you generally want to have food that is low in acidity food and high in insoluble fiber. Therefore, if your stools are lacking volume you should eat more vegetables, fruits, legumes, nuts and seeds. Here are some foods that I highly recommend for increasing stool volume: Bananas, avocados, green beans, turnip, sweet potatoes, yams, beans, chickpeas, lentils, and whole grains. These are great food for increasing volume because they are easy on the digestive system and are relatively low in acidity, therefore you can eat a lot of them.

Stool Stickiness

Stool stickiness can go two ways. First, your stools may be too sticky, as indicated by overly hard and tight stools. Second, your stools may be not sticky enough as indicated by stools that easily fall apart and do not form together.

Excessively Sticky Stools: The treatment for excessively sticky stools is to reduce dairy and meat intake (especially red meat, if excessive) and increase moisture and volume of your stools. To do this, drink more water and follow the guidelines in the stool volume section.

Non-Sticky Stools: The treatment for non-sticky stools is to increase intake of food that is easy to digest, high in starch content, oily, and contains probiotics. Here is a list of food you should consider: Easy to digest and starch rich food like bananas, rice, spaghetti, cooked vegetables, eggs, oats, and well-cooked whole grains. Oily food like olive oil, coconut oil, almond oil, unsweetened peanut butter, cashew butter, and chia and flax seeds. Fermented food like kimchi, natto, miso, pickled food, sauerkraut, low fat yogurt, and chutneys. You can also supplement with probiotics if you do not have access to any fermented food that works well with your stomach.

Note that your stools may also be falling apart easily if you mainly eat fruit and vegetables. If this is your case, you should substitute for a more wholesome diet that includes whole grains, legumes, nuts, seeds, healthy root vegetables, and animal products.

Easy Fiber

Getting enough fiber can be difficult. So, here are some suggestions for easy fiber: Try psyllium seed husk fiber, ground flax seed meal, chia seeds, have easy to access fruits and vegetables handy (e.g. bananas, dried prunes, pre-washed vegetables, keep a pre-washed fruit and vegetable bowel, etc.), keep nuts and seeds handy, substitute processed grains for whole grains, etc.

Note that if you increase your fiber intake, it is also critically important that you also increase your water intake by either drinking more liquids or eating more water rich foods.

Fermented Food

Fermented food is rich in probiotics that boost immunity, fight gut inflammation, help with food digestion, and alleviate many digestive abnormalities. This makes them very effective for alleviating the nutcracker syndrome. Probiotics include kefir, buttermilk, natto, miso, tempeh, kimchi, sauerkraut, cheese, low fat yogurt, chutney, etc. You should have some fermented food daily. As well, you I recommend testing to change the fermented food that you eat for at least one month to see if it makes a difference on your bowel or digestive health.

Supplements

Vitamin D: Vitamin D is critically important for bowel and overall health. Unless you are getting 5 (pale white skin) to 20 minutes (black skin) of direct sun exposure daily, you need to be supplementing with Vitamin D.

Probiotics: There are many probiotics, and each have various benefits and effects on the body. You should test out different probiotics supplements if you have bowel or digestive problems. You can consult a qualified healthcare practitioner to learn more.

NORMAL AMOUNT OF SALT

High salt levels cause many symptoms that are bad for your varicocele. For example, high salt levels cause bacteria in the stomach to deteriorate the stomach lining, leading to inflammation. Salt also slows down digestion by interfering with digestive enzyme secretion. It can also dehydrate stools, causing constipation. Moreover, it increases blood pressure and viscosity. And can cause water retention and swelling.

Note: I am not saying stop having salt in your diet. Salt is critical for bodily functions. I am saying normalize your salt intake; do not intake excessive amounts of salt.

FERTILITY

There are many herbs, roots, powders, supplements, and dietary changes that can help significantly improve fertility. I cover just three here, but you can visit my website for a comprehensive review of all of the best natural remedies for improving fertility.

More Fertility Nutrition Advice: For more tips on what food and supplements aid in fertility, visit the resource page of my website. varicocelehealing.com/fertility-treatment

Carnitine, L-Carnitine & L-Acetylcarnitine: Carnitines are naturally occurring compounds found in the human body, they have many benefits for fertility. They are a potent antioxidant that provide protection against reactive oxygen species (major cause of infertility in men with varicocele). Supplementation with carnitines helps improve sperm count, concentration, motility, morphology, maturation, and prevent sperm DNA damage. Furthermore, they provide benefits for those suffering from asthenozoospermia, improve pregnancy rates, and may have beneficial effects for epididymitis.

The most prominent source of carnitines is red meat, but carnitines are also found in poultry, fish, and dairy products. Fruits, and vegetables carry minimal amounts.

Coenzyme Q10: A is naturally occurring compound and antioxidant present in most human cells. Coenzyme Q10 helps improve sperm count, concentration, motility, and morphology. It also lowers FSH and LH levels, and improves the success rate of pregnancy and in vitro fertilization.

Coenzyme Q10 is found in fish, organ meats (heart, kidney, and liver), nuts, soybeans, grains, and vegetables (i.e., cabbage, carrots, onions, potatoes, spinach, etc.)

Lycopene: Is a naturally occurring antioxidant with benefits for fertility. Infertile men have lower levels of lycopene than fertile men. Lycopene helps improve sperm count, concentration, motility, and morphology. Evidence also suggests that it helps improve pregnancy rates in those with sperm count of at least 5 million/mL.

Lycopene is found in tomatoes and other red fruits such as watermelon, grapefruit, red carrots, grapes, and papaya. Food that is not red may also contain lycopene, such as asparagus and parsley.

MORE TOPICS

Topics like normalizing testosterone production, improving prostate health, and enhancing sexual function with diet and nutrition are beyond the scope of this book. If you want to learn more on these topics, you can visit our learning center:

varicocelehealing.com/learning-center

CHAPTER DEFINITIONS

Anti-Inflammatory: Chemicals or treatments that reduce inflammation.

Antioxidants: Chemicals that disable oxidants.

Inflammation: A condition where a part of the body becomes red, swollen, hot, and often painful.

Oxidants and Reactive Oxygen Species (ROS): Chemicals that are harmful for sperm and fertility.

Stool: Feces.

Transit Time: The amount of time it takes for food to pass through the digestive system and be excreted.

Vasculoprotective Agent: A substance that protects the veins from damage.

Vein Contractility: The ability of the veins to squeeze and become thinner.

Venous Tonifying Agent: A substance that improves vein health, energy and strength.

CHAPTER 6

FITNESS & EXERCISES

CAUTION

Do Not Stop Being Active
All too often, doctors tell their patients with varicocele to completely stop all physical activity for a few weeks. This is a complete mistake. First off telling this to varicocele patients confuses and depresses them. Moreover, even though inactivity may potentially temporarily reduce varicocele symptoms, it comes with a host of other problems that are not healthy for varicocele and that will soon worsen varicocele symptoms. In this guide, you are given much more effective symptom management strategies than simply stopping all activities.

High Stress Activities
Ideally, you should supplement high stress activities with more therapeutic ones. This will help improve your treatment results. Note that I am not saying you should stop the high stress activities completely.

Be cautious of high stress activities that are jumping focused, highly strenuous, overheating for the testicles, and cause physical trauma to the testicles and testicular veins.

Jumping Focused: E.g. Basketball, volleyball, etc.

Highly Strenuous: E.g. Weightlifting, martial arts, sprinting, etc.

Overheat the Testicles: E.g. Long-distance running, biking, etc.

Cause Physical Trauma: E.g. Bicycling, horseback riding, etc.

Minimize High Stress Activity for 2 Weeks

Now, I am not saying stop being active completely or strop the all high stress activities forever. I am however saying that for your first two weeks of treatment, you need to treat your testicles and testicular veins as if they are injured and very sensitive. You therefore want to minimize stress on them by minimizing the amount of high stress physical activity that you perform for the first two weeks of treatment.

Notice that this does not mean stop being active. It does however imply that you should substitute high stress activities for healthier and more therapeutic ones, for the first two weeks. You may resume your high stress activities after two weeks.

THERAPEUTIC ACTIVITIES FOR VARICOCELE

To help enhance your varicocele treatment results, and improve your overall health, you should be performing some regular activity that is healing & meditative, promotes digestive health, has minimal vertical loading, stimulates cardiovascular health, develops posture, and/or alleviates tension from the hips.

HEALING & MEDITATION

Examples Include: Yoga, Tai Chi, Qi Gong, etc.

Healing & meditative activities put the body into the healing state, help promote healthy blood flow to the testicles, remove toxic stress from the body, stimulate the immune system, and boost digestive function, all at the same time as improving wellbeing and fitness. Everyone should perform some form of healing and meditative practice.

Meditation & Deep Breathing

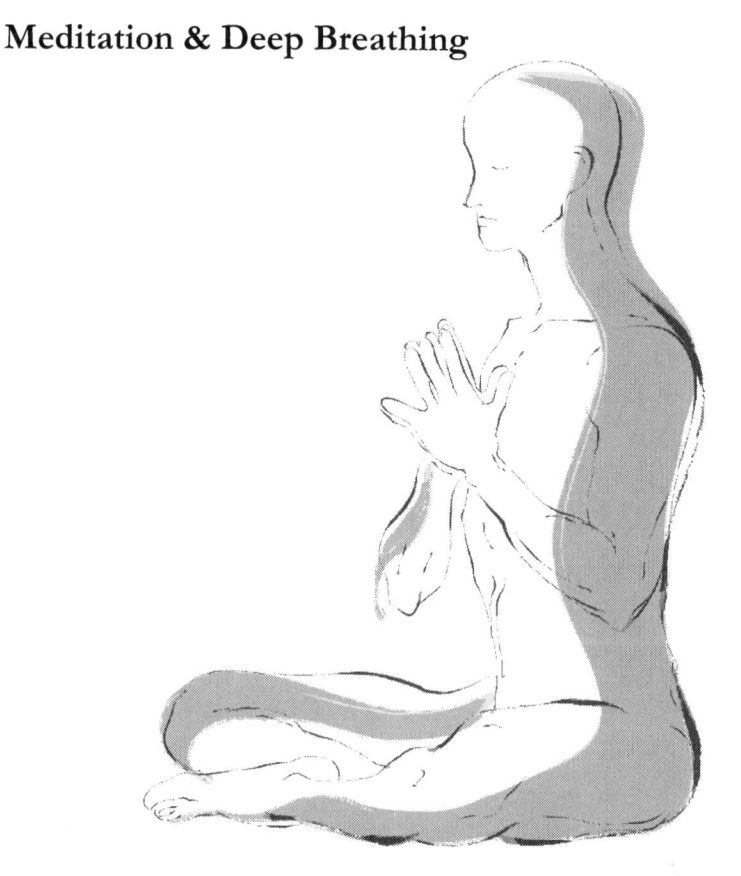

If you have a high stress lifestyle or are always in a rush, meditation and deep breathing can bring some well needed balance to your life and at the same time help improve your treatment results. Meditation and deep breathing promote relaxation, calm the body and mind, induce a meditative state, stimulate & activate the healing systems, strengthen and tone the digestive and vascular organs, and alleviate excessive pressure from the abdomen.

PROMOTE DIGESTIVE & ABDOMINAL HEALTH

Examples Include: Walking, light jogging, swimming, Yoga, etc.

Abdominal health is critical for varicocele treatment. Poor abdominal health typically results in more severe and persistent symptoms. Therefore, to improve treatment results, it is important to move, stimulate, and strengthen the abdominal muscles and organs.

The best activities for promoting digestive and abdominal health are those that involve forward, backward, and side bends, twists, inversions, and digestive specific exercises. Furthermore, up and down motions from walking, in and out motions from breathing, and various massaging techniques also promote digestive health.

Swimming is very good for improving digestive health. It bends, twists, stretches, and compresses the core, making it a unique and very healthy activity for digestive health.

Walks and light jogs are especially healthy for varicocele because they massage the digestive organs, stimulate bowel and lymph movement, and boost the immune system. For optimal bowl health, I recommend walking about 4-5 km total, daily.

Yoga has many poses, inversions, breathing techniques, and movements that help stimulate and promote digestive health. Yoga is also very relaxing and meditative, and promotes the rest, digest, and healing state. These make yoga a very healthy activity for varicocele treatment.

Crunches

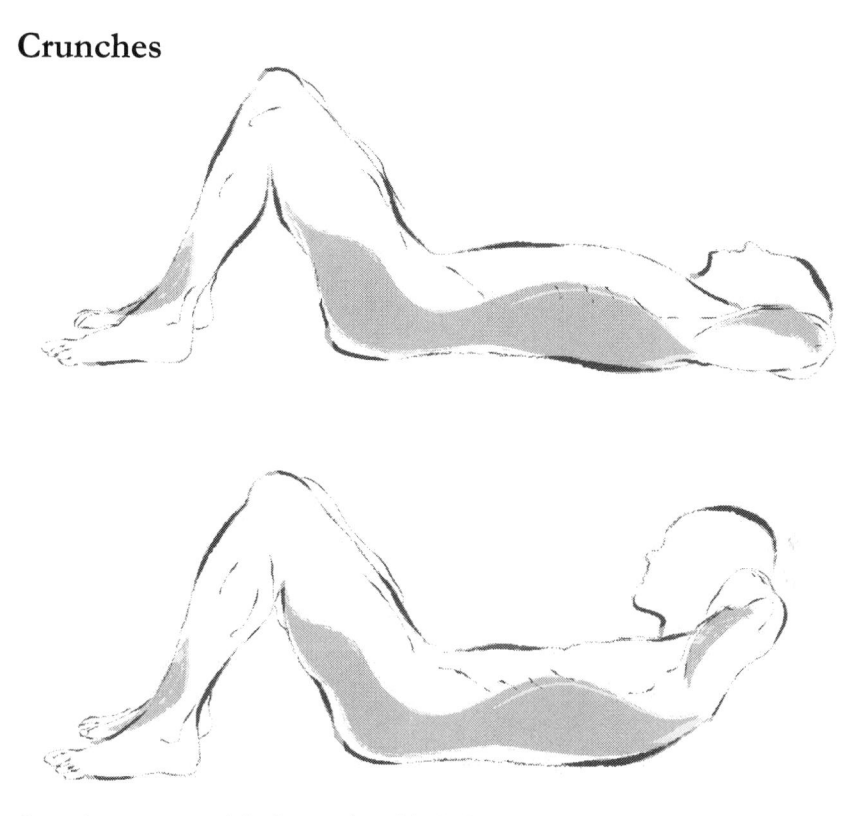

Crunches are a straightforward and helpful exercise. They squeeze your navel area and help increase abdominal strength and massaging your digestive organs.

Begin by lying on your back with your knees bent. Your feet should be about as wide as your hips. Place your hands behind your head so your thumbs are underneath your ears and your fingers are on the back of your head. Exhale and curl up and forward, so that your head, neck, and shoulder roll off the floor. Pause for a moment at the top, then slowly inhale and un-curl; lowering back to the ground. That is one repetition.

This is a simple and easy exercise to perform. Anyone can do it. I recommend performing at least 10 repetitions daily.

Caution: This is not a neck exercise; your neck should remain in-line with your torso throughout the exercise. Make sure you do not pull your head forward with your hands.

Reverse Crunches

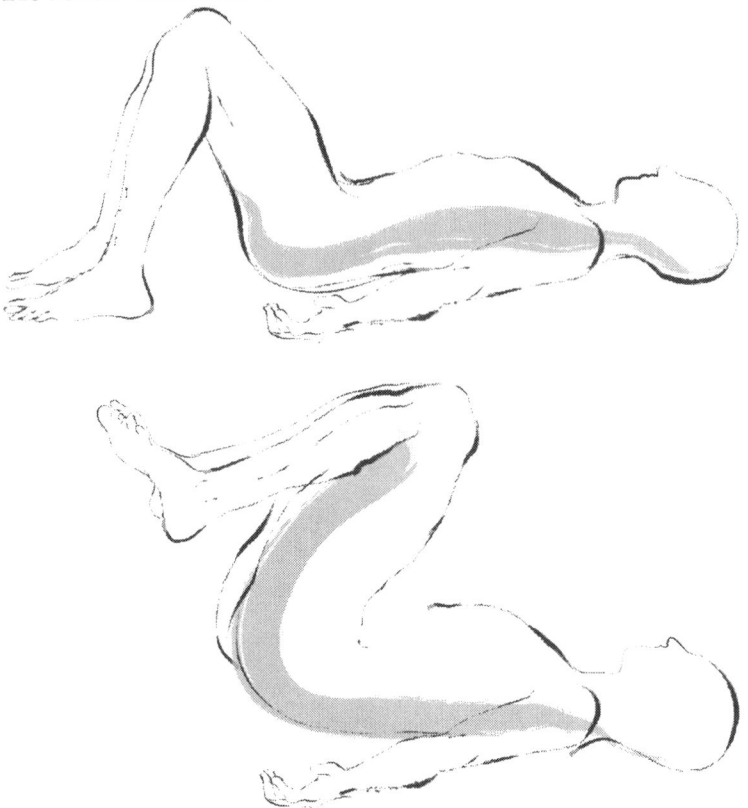

The reverse crunch is great for strengthening and toning the lower abdominal belt. The lower abdominal belt helps minimize pressure in the lower torso. This makes it beneficial for varicocele that results from sitting all day, having a weak core, or poor posture. Flexing and stimulating the lower abdomen also helps alleviate flatulence, stimulate bowel movement, prevent bowel inflammation, and promote bladder emptying. This makes it very healthy for varicocele.

Note: Increasing the strength of the lower abdomen is critical for long-term varicocele treatment.

Begin laying on your back with bent knees. Brace your lower back by flattening your lower back on the ground. Now, lift your feet up to begin the exercise. Slowly straighten your legs slightly. Then ben and curl your legs back over your abdomen. For optimal results, perform at least 10 slow repetitions daily.

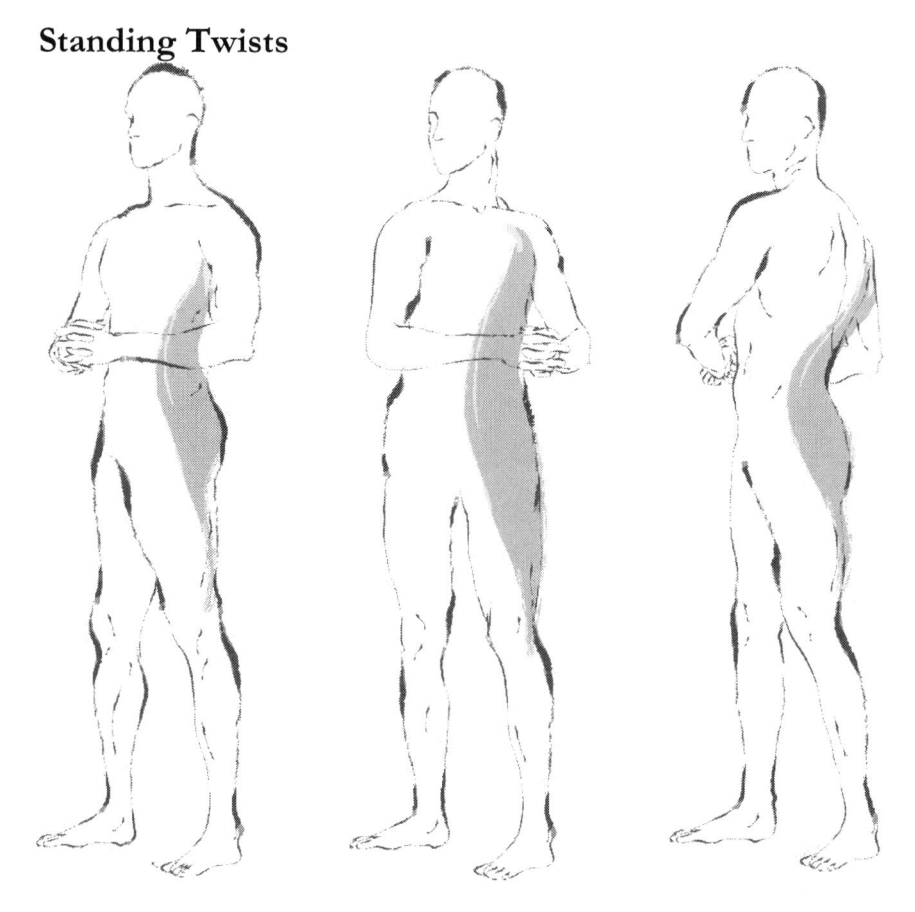

Standing Twists

Twisting in the mornings is a great way to stimulate bowel movement, develop a set bowel movement schedule, and strengthen the core muscles.

Begin by standing with your legs shoulder width apart. Keep your knees slightly bent. Now twist from one side to another. Exhale when twisting, and inhale when unwinding.

The closer your arms are to your body, the easier this exercise is. Your goal is therapy. Therefore, it is okay and recommended to perform this exercise at low intensity.

Note: Do not perform twists on a full or bloated stomach.

Diamond Belly Rub

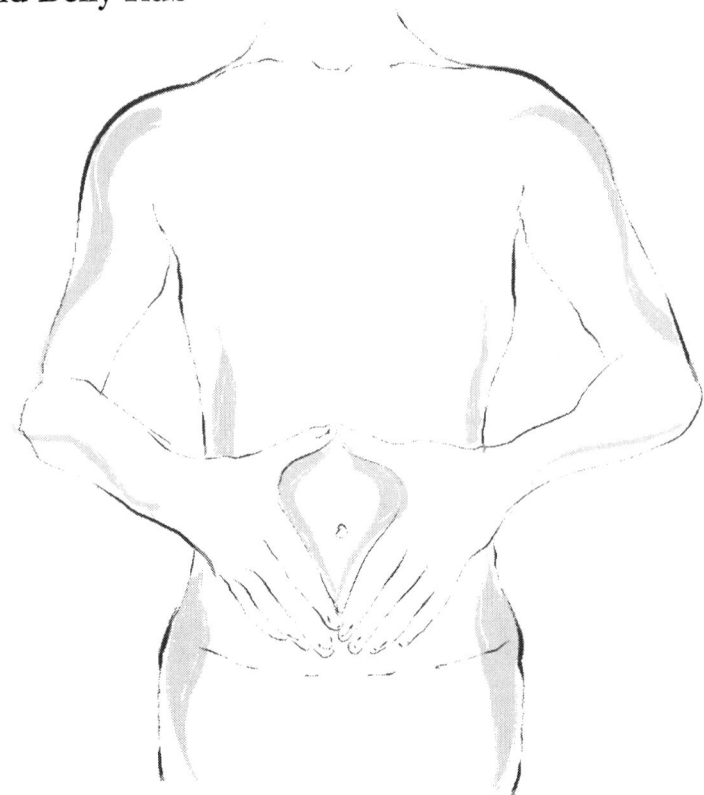

When you wake up in the morning, rubbing your belly can be very stimulating for bowel movements and promote lymph drainage. This is a gentle massage that aids in developing a set bowel movement schedule and is also good for improving bowel and digestive health.

Perform this exercise when standing. Make a diamond shape by touching your index fingers and thumps together. Begin gently rubbing your belly with your palms. Massage in circles around, but not over, your belly button.

Perform at least 10 clockwise and counterclockwise circles. Ideally perform this exercise every morning.

Note: This is a gentle exercise, perform it with calmness of mind. Do not press into your abdomen. Your goal is to heat up, gently massage and stimulate blood flow to the area, not to irritate your intestines.

Jumping / Rebounding

Jumping/rebounding is great for digestive health. It massages the internal organs and is great for constipation. Jumping activities also help promote hormone balance, and the drainage of stagnant mucus and lymph.

Simply stand in one spot and jump up and down or use a rebounder. You do not have to jump high; it is enough for your feet to just leave the ground. Use your try to use feet, knees, and hips for jumping and landing. Keep the exercise light. Jump 25 times every other morning.

Caution: Please take the following precautions before performing jumping/rebounding activities as a form of therapy for varicocele:

Good Posture: Make sure to perform jumping/rebounding activities with good posture (no collapsed chest or protruding lower abdomen).

Pre-Activity Cooling: Perform a cooling treatment before the activity (e.g. run cold water over your testicles for 10-15 seconds).

Not When Swollen: Do not perform jumping/rebounding activity if your varicocele is swollen or if it worsens your symptoms. You must also perform a cooling treatment before you begin the exercise.

Limit Time: Limit these activities to 2-5 minutes per day.

Minimal Intensity: Perform with minimal intensity.

Proper Core Activation: For proper core activation, do not perform these activities on a full or un-bloated stomach.

Standing Forward Bends

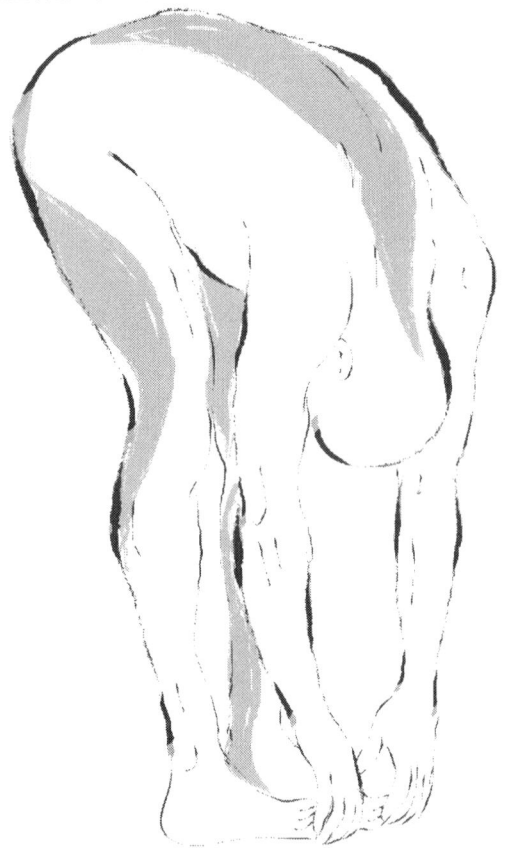

Inversion exercises, including the standing forward bend, are generally very good for toning and removing toxicity from the digestive organs, and alleviating flatulence and constipation.

Start this exercise by standing with your legs about hip width apart. Keep a small bend in your knees. Now, simply bend forward and hold the bottom position for 10 to 20 seconds. Make sure to inhale and exhale fully.

Note: If the intensity of this pose is too high, increase the bend of your knees, or rest one or both arms your thighs.

MINIMAL VERTICAL LOAD (MVL)
Examples Include: Swimming, Yoga, rock climbing, etc.

Because excessive vertical loading is associated with both varicocele development and severity, it is critical for us to perform more MVL activities. Moreover, MVL activities are a beneficial for both health and improving fitness, but, they do not get the recognition that they deserve. It should be noted that almost all therapeutic, meditative, and healing activities are minimal vertical loading activities. High vertical loading activities used to be a necessity for survival, but now, we have the option of supplementing with activities that are more health promoting.

Swimming is a form of MVL activity. Your body is normally horizontal when you swim, therefore it has negligible vertical loading. Furthermore, being submerged in water means that the water pressurizes your body, further reducing vertical load and making venous drainage easier. This is not to mention all the other great benefits of swimming.

Yoga is also great form of MVL activity, because it understands the value of activities that involve inversions, lying down, spinal decompression, and minimal vertical strain. Unfortunately, most yoga poses and classes are far too advanced for new and even regular practitioners.

Rock climbing and other forms of pulling-self-up activity (e.g. pull-ups, gymnastics, etc.) are also noteworthy because they combine decompression with physical activity.

CARDIOVASCULAR HEALTH
Examples Include: Jogging, swimming, elliptical, etc.

Cardiovascular activity is important because it improves vein contractility, tone, and health. Furthermore, cardiovascular activity helps normalize blood pressure, and reduce resting blood pressure and heart rate.

Some people make the mistake of strengthening and building only their muscles, without developing the foundation—their cardiovascular health. This is not a good approach because with muscle development comes increased metabolic demand and cardiovascular output for maintenance.

Any activity that elevates your heart rate for at least 10 to 15 minutes continuously and makes you sweat is a form of cardiovascular activity. Some good forms of cardiovascular activity include jogging, swimming, and using the elliptical machine.

DEVELOP MUSCLE BALANCE & POSTURE

Examples Include: Educated strength training, gymnastics, etc.

Poor muscle balance and posture (e.g. forward head posture, anterior pelvic tilt, posterior pelvic tilt, asymmetric postures, etc.) are major contributing factors to varicocele development and severity. They are discussed in further detail later in this chapter.

Salutation Pose:

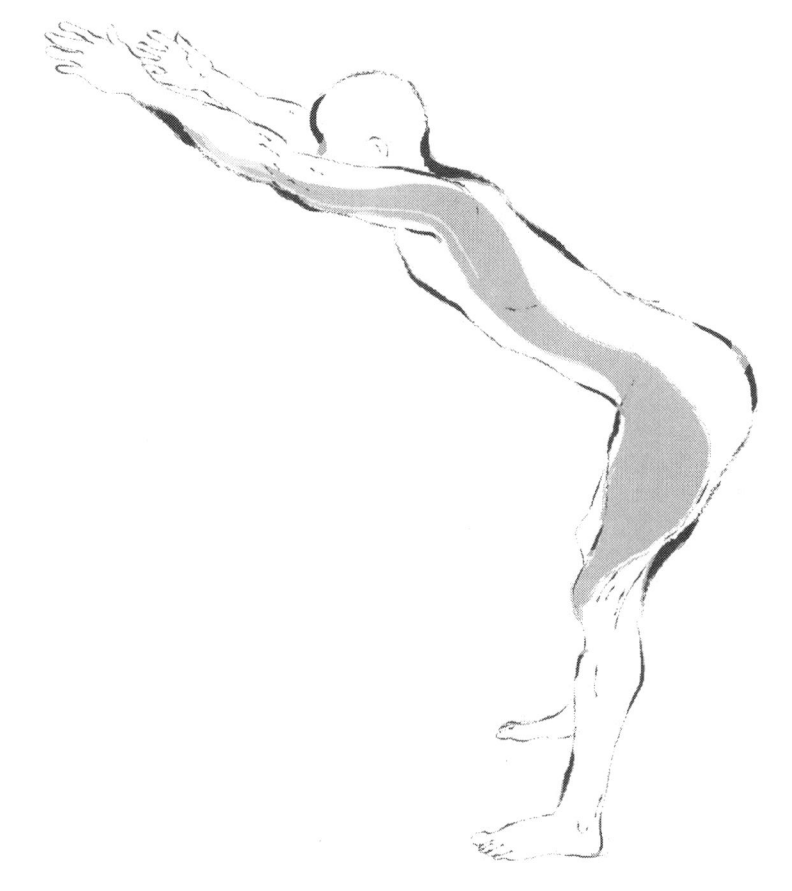

The salutation pose is a great pose for strengthening the entire posterior chain, making it a great exercise for developing healthier posture.

Start by standing with your feet about shoulder width apart. From here, bend forward by pushing back and hinging from your hips. Keep a neutral arc in the lower back; do not bend from the lower back. Maintain a very minimal and slight bend at the knees. Keep bending until you get to about 45 degrees. Hold this position for a moment. Now sweep your arms up from your sides to above your head. Keep your arms straight. Your goal is to from a straight line with your arms and body.

Hold this position for 5-20 deep breaths. Perform daily.

ALLEVIATE TENSION FROM HIPS
Examples Include: Yoga, stretching, etc.

Everyone can benefit from the occasional stretching and loosening up. The benefits include improved blood circulation, muscle balance, range of motion, reduced joint stress and muscular tension, etc. Moreover, stretching and loosening up can all be beneficial for varicocele, especially for those who lead a sedentary lifestyle and those who are overly active.

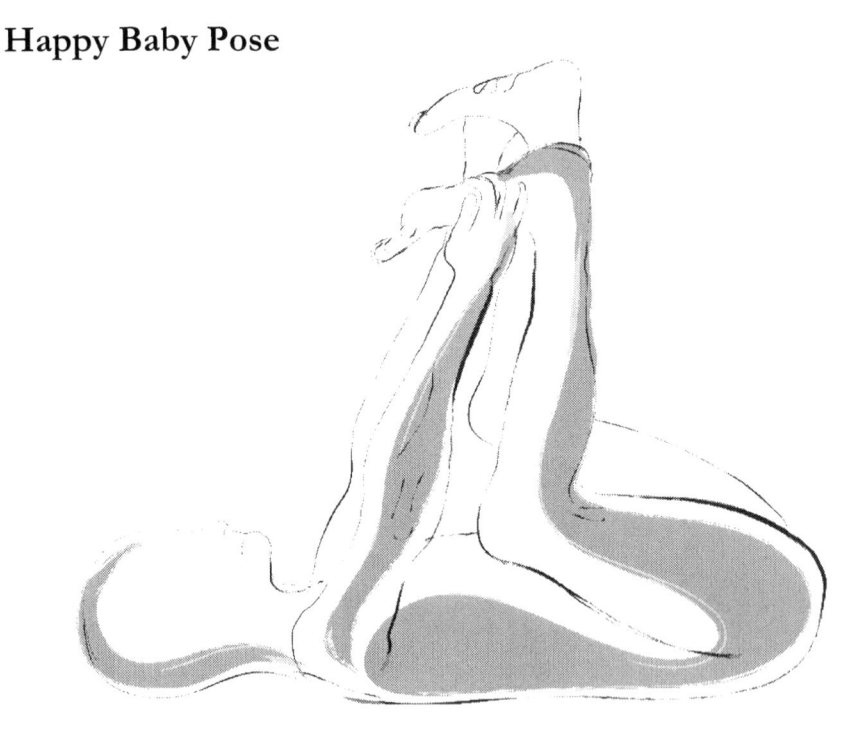

Happy Baby Pose

The happy baby pose is another one of my favorite exercises. It is very easy to perform, hold for long periods, and has great benefits. It is a mild inversion exercise, and therefore has the added benefit of draining the varicocele. It also stretches and tones the pelvic floor, reducing muscular tension, and improving the blood circulation of in lower torso. It is especially important for bikers, runners, and anyone who sits or stands for prolonged periods.

Perform this exercise by lying on your back with your knees bent. Now, draw your knees up towards your chest. Grab the outsides of your feet with your hands and slowly draw your legs down until you attain a mild stretch. Do not roll your lower back off the floor when performing this exercise. Instead, try keeping your lower back relatively flat on the floor. Perform this pose every night for at least 30 seconds before sleep.

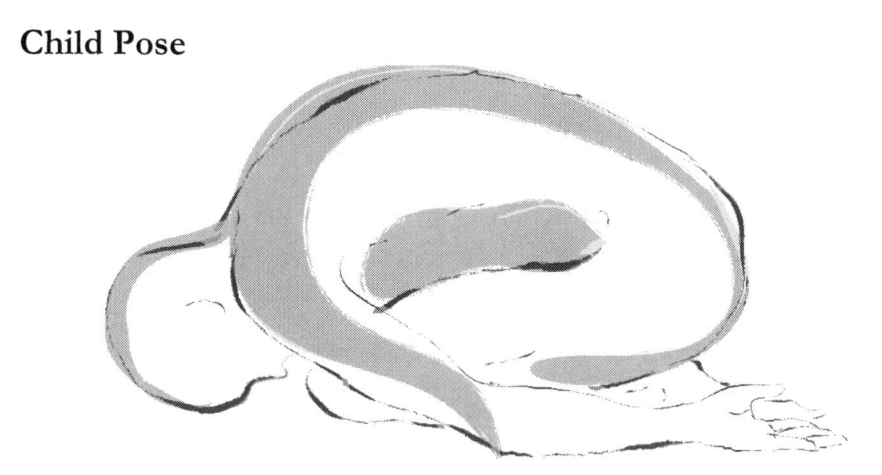

Child Pose

Child's pose is a great way to calm the mind and relax the body. It helps alleviate tension from and loosen up the hips. Furthermore, it is also therapeutic and easy to perform.

Start by sitting on your shins with the top of your feet on the ground. You can spread your knee as much as is comfortable. Slowly lower your head to the ground or onto a pillow. Allow your arms to relax down by your sides. Now, hold this position for a 1-5 minutes. Perform every day.

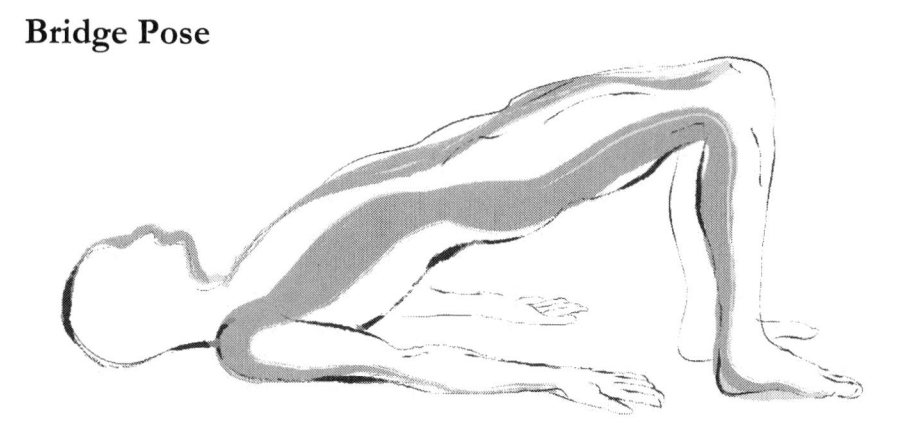

Bridge Pose

The bridge pose is a great exercise for opening the hips up after a long day of sitting. It also helps strengthen the posterior chain (hamstrings, glutes, and spinal erectors), and is an inversion exercise so it has the added benefit of draining the varicocele and promoting digestion.

Begin laying on your back. From here bend your knees to where is comfortable (you can adjust your feet position at any time). Now, push your hips up until your thighs, hips and torso make a straight line. You can hold this position or raise the hips up higher. Hold this pose for 30 seconds or more. You may progress to holding the position for 5-10 minutes.

Note: You can alleviate pain or tension in the neck by facing your palms completely up, and then pulling them down towards your legs.

ACTIVE WITH VARICOCELE

People that are more active have a higher chance of developing varicocele—but, people who are less active typically have higher incidence of infertility and disease. Sounds a bit confusing right? Just think of it this way: Activity is good for fertility and varicocele. However, if you only perform high stress activities, take no preventative measures, and do not perform the activities with caution, then you are likely doing more damage than good. So, here, we have a ton of tools that we can use to make our activities therapeutic, and less damaging.

General Advice

Pre-Workout Cooling: A cooling treatment (e.g. running cold water over your testicles and varicocele for 15 second, etc.) before activity can help stimulate contraction of the varicose veins, and pull the scrotum up to pressurize the scrotum. This reduces varicocele swelling size, provides natural compression, and protects against genital heat stress (is especially effective if you continue to keep your scrotum cool during activity). This is ideal for all forms of activity, but is especially useful for high intensity & jumping activities like martial arts, weightlifting, basketball, volleyball, etc.

Keep Cool During Activity: Most forms of activity overheat the testicles because they must be performed with underwear and pants on. Therefore, there is typically an inadequate heat ventilation during activity. Overheating increases varicocele swelling (in a dysfunctional attempt to cool the testicles) and makes the scrotum hang lower. Therefore, to mitigate activity risk factors, and for varicocele treatment, and symptom recovery, it is critical to ensure that your testicles do not overheat during activity. This is especially important for you if you spend many hours a week being active.

Post-Activity Cooling: A cooling treatment (e.g. 1-2 minutes under cool water) after activity is great for reducing inflammation and promoting recovery. I recommend it for everyone with varicocele.

Workout Attire! Not Tight & Breathes Well: Proper workout attire will help make your workouts more therapeutic than stressful. Do not wear pants or underwear that are excessively tight or have excessively tight waists. As well, try to wear pants and underwear that breathe well.

Activate and Loosen Up Hips: Modern lifestyles typically tightens up and weakens the hips. Tight hips increase the tension in daily activities and transfer the tension to the core and other parts of the body. This is non-ideal for varicocele. So, you should stretch regularly! Furthermore, weak hips mean poor posture and improper mobility. It helps to time on spent on hip activation pre- or post-workout.

Post-Workout Stretching: A post-workout stretch routine is effective for allowing the body to remove toxins, reducing blood toxicity, boosting recovery, and helping relax and re-place the body into the healing state. It is healthy and beneficial for varicocele treatment to perform post-workout stretches.

Post-Activity Inversions: An inversion post-workout boosts workout recovery and can help prevent worsening of varicocele symptoms associated with stressful activities. You can simply put your legs up on a wall, or lay on your back with your knees bent, perform the bridge pose, or even a shoulder stand. Choose whatever inversion you like and hold it for a total time of 1 to 5 minutes.

Technique Advice
Axial Extension (Beginner):

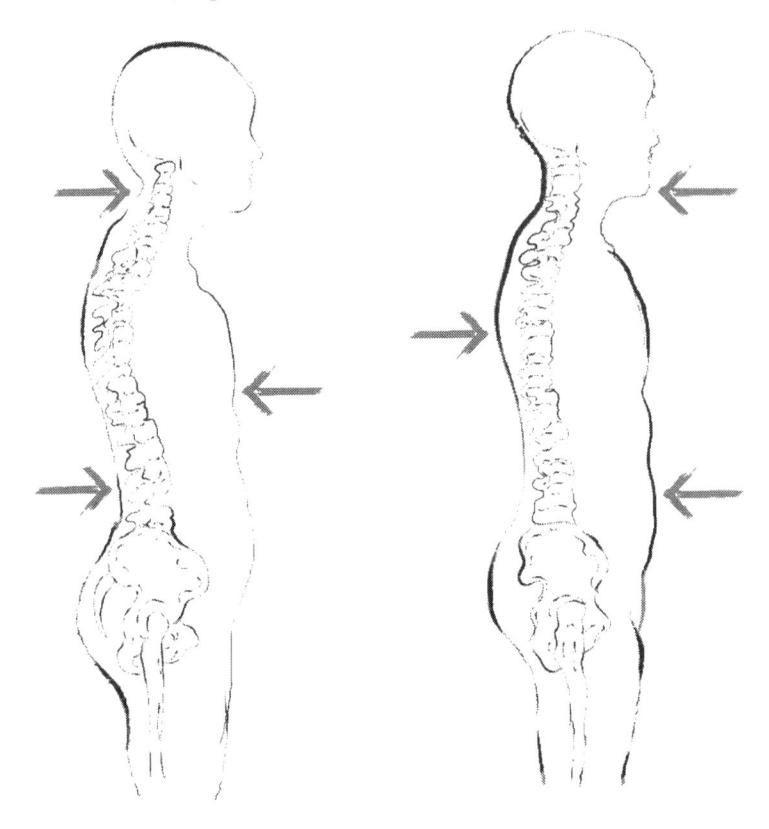

The axial extension exercise is very important for improving posture and minimizing stress on your varicocele during strenuous activity. It is a common technique practiced in almost all sports and yoga. The exercise lengthens your torso, shifting the weight from the varicocele and digestive organs to the core and spinal muscles.

Even though this is beginner bracing sequence, it is foundational for posture, and is one of my favorite exercises because it is so easy, can be performed anytime and during any activity, and has many benefits.

Simply put, the axial extension exercise is lengthening the torso and neck into better alignment. To perform it, reach for the ceiling with the crown of your head and for the floor with your hips. You should feel a nice stretch in your torso. Your chin should tuck in slightly you should feel a stretch in the back of your neck. Don't forget to keep breathing normally.

It is critically important to perform an axial extension when carrying heavy loads (e.g., when wearing a heavy backpack, lifting weights at the gym, carrying groceries, etc.)

Note: The goal is to lengthen and normalize the spinal arcs.

Proper Technique (Advanced): Proper technique is more than just the beginner axial extension. More advanced technique requires video or in person instructions to learn. You can use the following key terms to search online for advanced technique: Core bracing, back bracing, proper breathing technique, hamstring loading, glute activation, hip flexor activation, knee stabilization, spinal stabilization, chin tuck, scapula mobility, scapula stabilization, and shoulder stabilization. As well, you should always search for technique specific to the activity you perform.

Breathing: During exercise, you typically want to exhale when you push against gravity (exerting) and inhale when moving with gravity. As well, you want to exhale when you do forward bends (flexing at the hips or abdominals), and inhale when unbending or stretching backwards (extending at the hips or abdominals).

The idea behind these breathing patterns is to strengthen your core, prevent unnecessary stress on your internal organs, and to minimize pressure build up in the lower torso when exerting. They also ensure that your internal organs move out of the way and are supported during activity.

Valsalva Maneuver (Advanced): Contrary to popular belief, it is okay for those who have varicocele to perform the Valsalva maneuver. It is however an advanced breathing technique. If you do perform the Valsalva maneuver make sure that you exert with proper technique and spinal alignment, good posture, maybe perform a pre-activity cooling treatment, and make sure that you have good bracing of your core and lower abs.

Biking: I recommend not biking if you have a varicocele. It is associated with increased incidence of varicocele and more severe varicocele symptoms. Biking causes microtrauma to the testicles and veins, tightens up the hip area, creates many muscle imbalances that are difficult to correct, is associated with genital heat stress, and is one of very few forms of activity that place very high pressure in the lower torso for long periods.

If you want to continue biking, I have several recommendations: Do not bike for excessively long periods (e.g., over 30 minutes per day). Do your best to bike on even ground to minimize vibrations that cause microtrauma to the veins and testicles. Do not wear underwear when biking, instead, wear only breathable shorts. Bike standing once in a while to allow proper heat exchange. Bike with good posture to reduce pressure on your lower torso. Ideally use a speed/road bike with a forward arm rest to minimize vertical loading. Do not use mountain bikes that force you into a vertical posture. Do not bike with a full or bloated stomach. Stretch your hips and pelvic floor after biking (e.g. with happy baby pose, bridge pose, etc.)

If you take the precautions outlined above, you can get away with biking for long periods. However, biking should be considered as an advanced from of activity because of the complexity of managing the precautions and correcting the tightness and muscular imbalances that it develops.

Running: Like biking, long-distance running is associated with varicocele development. I do not recommend running long-distance unless you take some precautions. Do not run on a full stomach or when bloated. Perform a cooling treatment pre- and post-running. Wear proper clothes that are not tight and allow proper heat ventilation. Stretch and warmup before running. Activate the hips, posterior chain, and core pre-running. Run with proper technique. Run with good posture. Stretch your hips post-running. Perform a 5-15 minute inversion post-running. Be cautious, maybe on a day that your varicocele is very swollen and painful, it is better to be patient and perform more therapeutic activities.

Running is an advanced activity. There are a ton of subtle technique changes that can make a big difference. If you have not already, you should research running technique.

Anaerobic (High-Intensity) Exercises: Those with varicocele should perform high-intensity activities with caution. Some examples of high-intensity activities are weightlifting, martial arts, and sprinting. High-intensity activities require short bursts of high effort. Performing high-intensity activities is important for overall health, but should be performed with caution to minimize risk.

I have almost the same advice for high-intensity activities as biking and running. In addition to the other advice given for activity, make sure to supplement high-intensity activity with at least some therapeutic activities, have extended warmups and cooldowns, give high priority to educated technique, make sure to breath fully and properly, and allow adequate time for post-activity recovery.

MUSCULAR & POSTURAL IMBALANCES (ADVANCED)

Muscular imbalances have a large contribution to varicocele development and severity. Three major muscular imbalances are at fault, namely, posterior pelvic tilt, anterior pelvic tilt, and forward head posture. All of these imbalances misalign your abdominal organs, aggravate the nutcracker effect, pressurize the lower abdomen, impair and increase tension of normal breathing, disable proper breathing technique, inhibit proper blood circulation, and increase blood toxicity. If you have muscular imbalances, your varicocele symptoms are unlikely to alleviate before you adequately address them.

Caution: Postural and muscular imbalances are not easy to spot by untrained eyes, and can also be very difficult to correct once identified. I recommend seeing a qualified healthcare practitioner for further instruction if you think that you may have some postural or muscular imbalance. A skilled personal trainer, physical therapist, and some general practitioners can be very helpful! I do offer personal training services that are specifically focused on varicocele treatment that you can take advantage of. My strategies and exercises are very effective both improving posture and varicocele treatment.

Anterior Pelvic Tilt (Advanced)

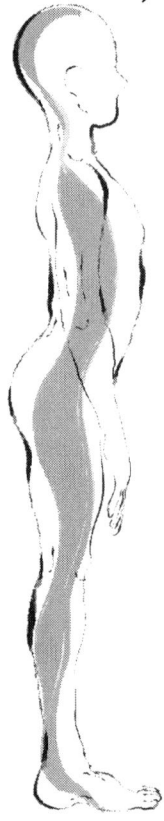

Anterior pelvic tilt is a postural imbalance. It means that the pelvis is tilted forward excessively. Think of it as the Donald Duck look—with the butt sticking out. It deactivates the abdominal muscles, pressurizes the lower abdomen, disables hip loading, and collapses the chest into the torso which pressurizes and impairs breathing.

Note: My presentation of the anterior pelvic tilt here is simplified and hip-centric. Anterior pelvic tilt can also be caused by non-hip factors.

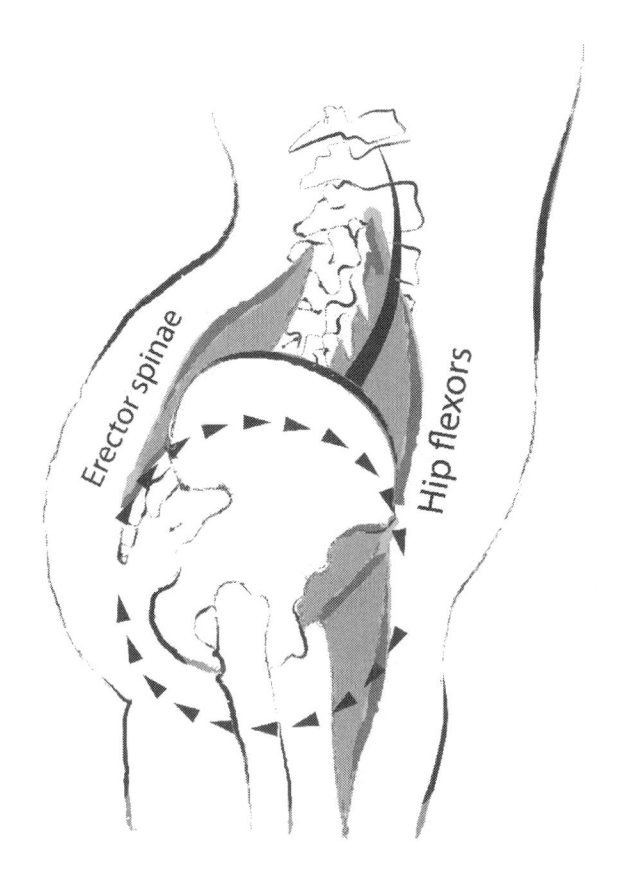

Anterior pelvic tilt is caused by tightness in and hyperextension of the lower back (hyperlordosis), and the forward tilting of the pelvis. This means that the following muscles are tight: Erector spinae, iliopsoas, and rectus femoris.

Therefore, to help correct your anterior pelvic tilt, you want to perform the following stretches: Child's pose to stretch and relax the erector spinae, standing or laying down quadriceps stretch, and a lunge stretch for the quadriceps and iliopsoas.

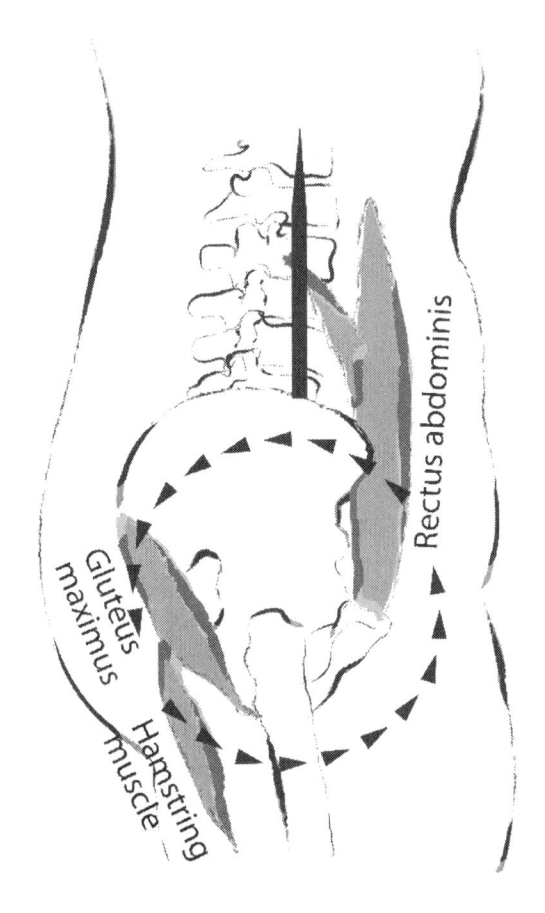

Anterior pelvic tilt is also caused by the inability of the hip to be pulled into a neutral alignment because of weak muscles. Weakness of the rectus abdominis enables the lower back to hyperextend, and weakness of the gluteus maximus and hamstrings enable the anterior pelvic tilt.

Therefore, to help correct your anterior pelvic tilt, you want to perform the following exercises: Crunches and reverse crunches to strengthen the rectus abdominis, and bridge pose to strengthen the glutes and hamstrings.

Posterior Pelvic Tilt (Advanced)

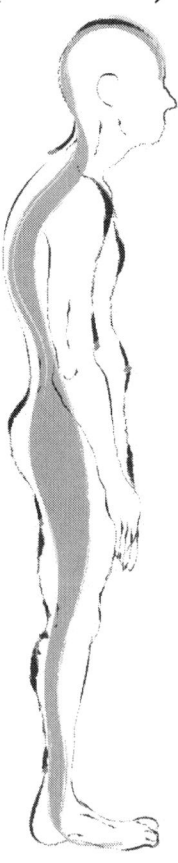

The posterior pelvic tilt is also a postural imbalance. It means that the pelvis is tilted backward excessively. Think of it as the Pink Panther look—with the butt tucked in and hips sticking forward. It deactivates, protrudes, and pressurizes the lower abdominals, collapses the chest into the abdominals which disables healthy breathing and pressurizes the abdominal organs, and deforms the spine and impairs proper hip mobility which also creates excessive load onto the abdominals.

Note: My presentation of the posterior pelvic tilt here is simplified and hip-centric. Posterior pelvic tilt can also be caused by non-hip factors.

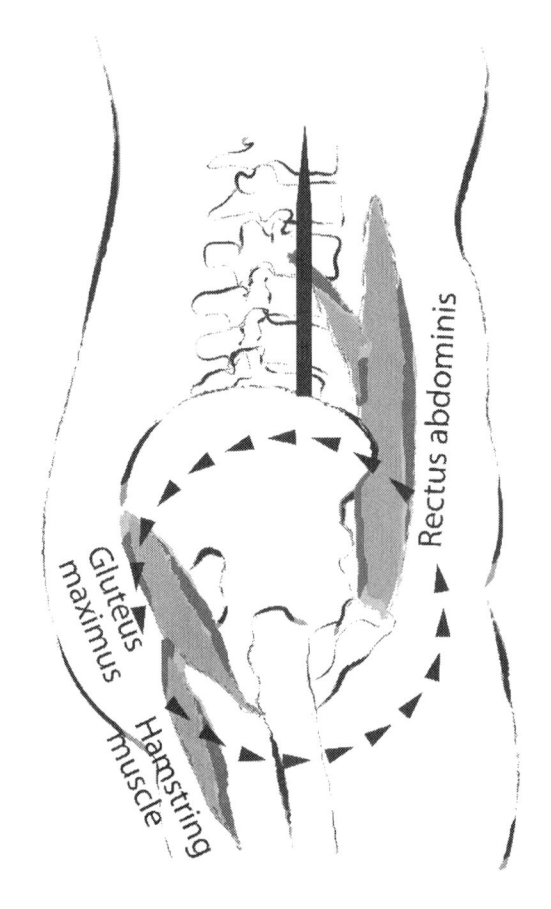

Posterior pelvic tilt is caused by excessive flexion of the lower back (hypolordosis), and the backward tilting of the pelvis. This means that the following muscles are tight: Rectus abdominis, glutes, and hamstrings.

Therefore, to help correct your posterior pelvic tilt, you want to perform the following stretches: Sphinx pose to help relax and stretch the abdominal muscles, pigeon pose to stretch the glutes, and forward reach to stretch the hamstrings.

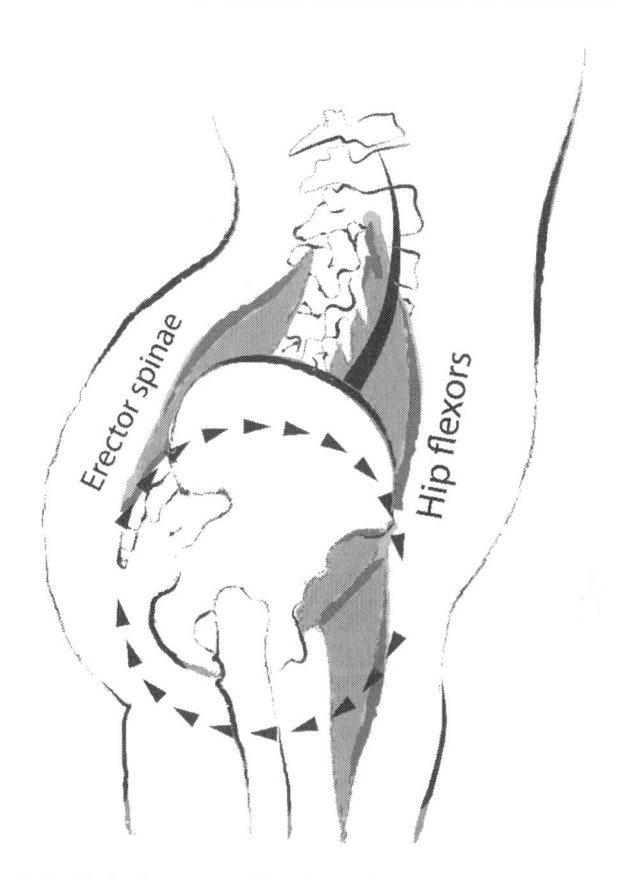

Posterior pelvic tilt is also caused by the inability of the hip to be pulled into a neutral alignment because of weak muscles. Weakness of the erector spinae enables excessive flexion of the lower back, and weakness of the iliopsoas and rectus femoris enable the posterior pelvic tilt.

Therefore, to help correct your posterior pelvic tilt, you want to perform the following exercises: Prone lower back extensions to strengthen the erector spinae, extended puppy pose to help strengthen the iliopsoas, and leg raises to strengthen the rectus femoris.

Forward Head Posture

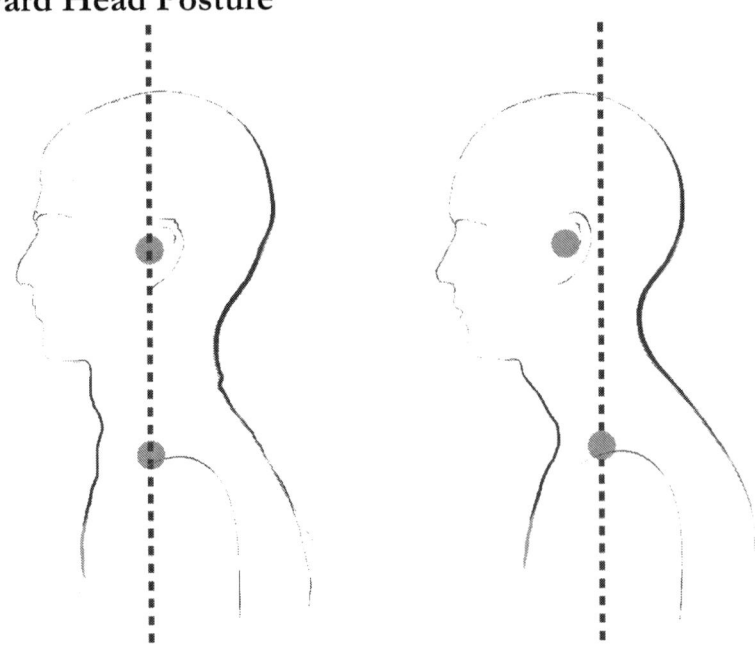

Forward head posture is a very common postural imbalance that negatively effects varicocele because it pulls the spine out of alignment. A misaligned spine impairs full and proper abdominal breathing, disrupts the integrity of the abdominal organs, and increases intra-abdominal pressure. These all contribute to higher incidence of varicocele and more severe symptoms.

Forward head posture is typically due muscular imbalances, namely, weak spinal erectors and hyoid muscles, and tight sternocleidomastoid muscles. We can correct these muscular imbalances with three exercises. The salutation pose strengthens the spinal erectors, and jaw opening exercise strengthens the hyoid muscles. The chin tuck exercise is very effective for specifically strengthen the neck spinal erectors and brining balance to tight sternocleidomastoid muscles.

Other Postural Imbalances (Advanced)

It is also important to mention that any asymmetric postures are also very unhealthy for varicocele. If one side of your shoulders or hips is elevated, or if you have scoliosis, you should consult a specialist.

CONSULT A PROFESSIONAL

Now, I know that this was likely a difficult chapter for many people. If you require further assistance or think that you have some condition that you do not fully understand, you should consult a healthcare professional. A high-quality professional can have a big positive impact on your treatment results.

Personal Trainer or Sports Therapist: If you need help with learning various exercises, proper training technique, improving your core health and strength, and correcting postural and muscular imbalances, you should seriously consider investing in a personal trainer or sports therapist.

You can visit my website to see if personal training is good option for you:

varicocelehealing.com/personal-trainer

Physiotherapist: Physiotherapists are typically more qualified and educated. They should be seen for taking care of more serious physical problems (e.g. persistent postural or muscular issues, spinal problems, joint pain, etc.)

CHAPTER DEFINITIONS

Anterior Pelvic Tilt: Hip tilting forward.

Forward Head Posture: The head being too far forward. It strains the entire length of the spine and pulls it out of optimal alignment.

Glutes: The main butt muscle.

Hamstrings: The main muscles at the back of the thighs.

Hip Flexors: Any muscle that lips your thighs up.

Muscle Imbalance: When muscles on one side of a joint are too strong when compared to the muscles on the opposing side.

Pelvic Tilt: The direction the hip tilts; forward or backward.

Pelvis: The hip bone.

Posterior Pelvic Tilt: Hip tilting backward.

Quadriceps: The main muscles at the front of the thighs.

Rectus Abdominis: The six-pack muscle.

Rectus Femoris: The quadriceps muscle that also flexes the hips.

DANIEL JOHNSON

CHAPTER 7

HEALING

CHAPTER INTRO

From my experience there are three steps to healing varicocele. First, you must alleviate varicocele induced stress and damage so your veins and testicles can actually recover. Then you must find out what factors specifically contribute to your case and remedy them. From there, you must perform some healing and therapeutic treatments to help stimulate healing of your varicocele.

For most people, many factors contribute to varicocele development and severity. I therefore highly advise reading over the entire guide and following as many of the treatments as possible. You should also be specific in your varicocele treatment. It is better to address the specific causes of your varicocele development instead of performing many general treatments.

ALLEVIATE VARICOCELE INDUCED DAMAGE & STRESS

The absolute first thing you need to do before you experience healing is to remove the stress and damage that is caused by varicocele. This means cool your testicles and circulate the blood. Refer to Chapter 2: Cooling & Pain Relief for cooling treatment. To counteract blood pooling, you must perform a minimum 10 minute inversion daily.

REDUCE BLOOD TOXICITY

High blood toxicity increases the damage to your veins and testicles and impairs healing. To reduce blood toxicity, you need to perform both dietary and lifestyle changes, for example, limit consumption of food that is highly processed, high in processed sugars, and that is highly acidic, make your diet less inflammatory, perform more light and medium intensity activity than high intensity activity, stop smoking and taking recreational drugs, limit drinking alcohol and coffee, manage and reduce your stress, etc.

INCREASE HEALTHY BLOOD FLOW

For healing you want less blood pooling, and more healthy blood flow to the testicles, veins, and surrounding tissue. To improve healthy blood flow, you can perform a testicle massage, penis stretch, massaging the inner thighs and perineum area (see Chapter 4: Fertility & Sexual Health) enter the healing state, breathe deeply, alleviate stress, take supplements such as Butcher's Broom, Grape Seed & Pine Bark, and vitamin K, attain erections, stretch and open up the hip muscles, and improving overall abdominal and digestive tone and health.

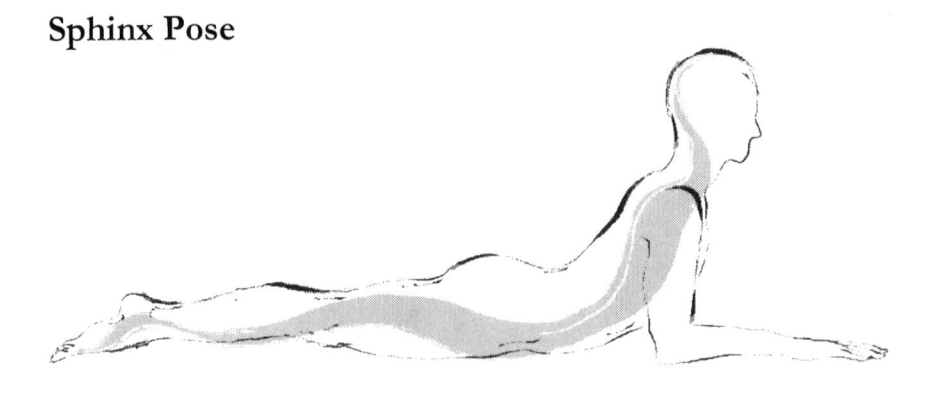

Sphinx Pose

The Sphinx pose is a great exercise for improving posture and increasing healthy blood flow to the digestive and reproductive organs. It is also an easy pose to hold for a several minutes.

Start by lying on your front. Place your elbows underneath your shoulders, push yourself up and raise your chest up. Your elbows should be directly underneath your shoulders. Support the weight of your torso with your shoulders and back muscles by pushing your arms firmly onto the ground. Do not allow your shoulders to shrug up. Keep your butt muscles tight to distribute the tension more evenly along your spine (i.e., do not put all the tension on your lower back).

I recommend performing this exercise every morning and holding it for at least 1-3 minutes.

VENOUS TONE

Veins have muscular and supportive tissue that surround them and aid in contraction, dilation, and venous emptying. Improving the muscle and tissue tone of the veins is therefore critical for healing, reducing the diameter of the blood vessels, and making them more resilient to pressure.

Cooling for Venous Tone

Cooling is an effective way of contracting and strengthening veins. When you begin the healing process, you should do some sort of cooling treatment daily to strengthen your veins. You can perform any cooling treatment, including cold showers, hot/cold water alternations, applying a cooling pack, etc. As you progress, however, you should not cool as often, but aim for normalizing scrotal temperatures instead (see Chapter 2: Cooling & Pain Relief for more details).

Nutrition for Venous Tone

Nutrition can be very effective for improving venous tone. Bilberries, bioflavonoids, Butcher's broom, gotu kola, horse chestnut seed, and vitamins B, C, E, & K are great. They contain specific chemicals that act as antioxidants (oxidative damage prevents healing of varicose veins and vein valves), alleviate venous inflammation, increases vein elasticity, protect venous connective tissue, tighten blood vessels, repair and maintain veins, enhance venous emptying, and have blood-thinning effects. See Chapter 6: Fitness & Exercises for further details.

Exercising for Venous Tone

Aerobic exercises are particularly important for stimulating venous strengthening and improving circulatory health. It is a good idea to regularly perform some form of aerobic activity. Ideally, perform non-jumping, non-abdominal-straining aerobic activities. Swimming and jogging are great options. See Chapter 6: Fitness & Exercises for more details.

Vein Massage

Caution: You must perform this treatment with caution. Only perform it before going to sleep at night and while in an inversion. You must perform a 5 minute inversion pre- and post- treatment. After your post- treatment inversion, you must perform a mild cooling treatment and then go to sleep. You must perform this treatment very gently. Do not perform if you have any other testicular or scrotal conditions other than varicocele.

That cautionary note aside, this treatment is safe. You may perform this treatment even if you have varicocele pain.

The vein massage treatment has many benefits. It helps loosen mildly tangled veins to stop pain to improve blood circulation and reduce excessive varicocele swelling. It can also stimulate vein strengthening and healing.

Begin this treatment in an inversion (e.g. legs up on wall). Now, gently grab your testicular veins between your middle and index fingers, and thumb. Lightly slip your fingers over the veins, rubbing at a 90 degree angle to the direction of your veins. Also feel along your veins and loosen up any mild tangling. Continue massaging for 1-2 minutes.

HEALING STATE

The healing state includes the rest and digest state, as well as specific stimulation of healing. It helps increase healthy blood flow to the testicles and testicular veins, reduce heart rate and blood pressure, remove blood toxicity, improve digestion, increase overall bodily wellbeing, and allows healing to occur.

Some great ways of stimulating the healing state are acupuncture, yoga, meditation, any mind-body practices, walking, stretching, laughing, quality sleep, napping, reducing blood toxicity, and deep abdominal breathing.

NUTCRACKER EFFECT

The nutcracker effect contributes greatly to varicocele swelling size. To reduce the nutcracker effect, you must improve your posture, digestive, bowel, and circulatory health, and improve your abdominal muscle tone. For posture, it is important to strengthen the posterior chain and stretch muscles that are tight from excessive sitting or to correct any imbalances that you may have from repetitive activity (see Chapter 6: Fitness & Exercises for more details). Digestive and bowel health are mainly improved by diet, stress management, and performing full torso inversions, exercises that stretch, bend and twist the torso, as well as abdominal breathing exercises. Circulatory health is mainly improved by diet and cardiovascular activity. Abdominal muscle tone is improved by general activity, core exercises, and toning the lower abdominal belt.

Abdominal Breathing

Generally, you want to breathe deeply with your stomach. When you inhale, your stomach should expand, and when you exhale, it should contract. This movement naturally massages your internal organs which improves lymph movement, digestive health, and blood circulation. Breathing deeply also nourishes the whole body with an adequate supply of oxygen and detoxifies and purifies the blood. Deep breathing also reduces stress and anxiety, putting the body into a healing state.

Breathing up in the lungs is very shallow. It also does not come with the same benefits of deep abdominal breathing. This is because deep breathing is linked to abdominal shape and is therefore highly connected to abdominal health.

I recommend practicing at least 5-10 minutes of deep breathing daily because it is very helpful varicocele healing. Moreover, you can practice it anytime and anywhere.

Creating Space in Abdominal Cavity

This exercise is very important for healing. It works by increasing space in the abdominal cavity, and shifts around your internal organs in a healthy way. For long-term healing, you must perform this exercise to help relieve the nutcracker effect. Ideally, perform it in the morning on an empty stomach.

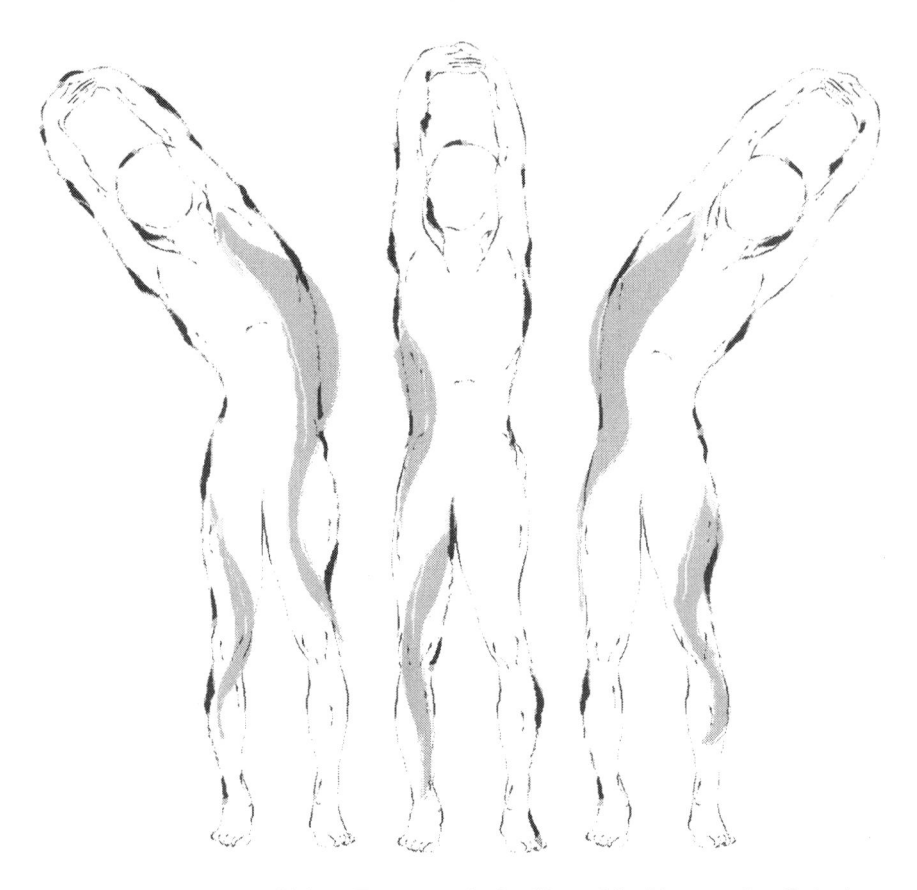

Reach Up & to the Sides: Everyone is familiar with this exercise. It is the same as yawning and stretching up. The exercise is an axial extension that also involves a deep diaphragm/abdominal breathing. It helps make room for venous drainage by shifting around your internal organs, and relieving built up abdominal tension and stress. It therefore helps treat the nutcracker effect, making it an important exercise for long-term healing.

Begin this exercise while standing. Exhale fully, and then reach up as high as you can with your arms. Keep your lungs empty and raise your chest up as you reach straight up and to the sides. You should note that as you raise your chest up, your navel pulls in and your digestive organs move upward. Hold the stretch for a moment, then inhale slowly as you relax down. Repeat five times straight up and five times to each side.

SCROTUM

Strengthening the cremaster muscle and preventing excessive scrotal sag is critically important for long-term healing. Excessive scrotal sagging occurs because the varicocele overheats and weighs down the scrotum. Over time, this stretches the cremaster muscle on the affected side. The lower the testicle hangs, the more blood pools, and a positive feedback mechanism initiates that increases the severity of the varicocele over time. Hanging low with pooled blood also tugs on your varicose veins and increases their susceptibility to damage. It can be the cause of pain. Therefore, it is important to provide support for the testicles and improve cremaster muscle tone.

Oil Massage: Note that an oil massage can help improve skin tone and have anti-inflammatory effects on the varicocele (see Chapter 4: Fertility & Sexual Health for more details.)

Providing Scrotal Support

You want to wear supportive underwear. Notice that I say support, and not compression. Compression abolishes the cremaster reflex and prevents testicular self-thermoregulation. Add this to the fact that varicocele already disrupts the cooling mechanism of the testicles and you end up with a lot of pain and testicular damage. So, do not wear excessively tight/compressive underwear. Refer to Chapter 2: Cooling & Pain Relief for more information.

Strengthening the Cremaster Muscle

You can strengthen your cremaster muscle with cooling treatments, erections, and self-flexion.

Cooling Treatments: Cooling treatments automatically activate the cremaster reflex. Over time, this is the most effective method for improving cremaster muscle tone.

Erections: Normally, the cremaster reflex accompanies erections. Therefore, healthy (and not excessive) masturbation, not necessarily with the point of orgasm, can be an effective method of strengthening your cremaster muscle and driving healthy blood flow to the testicles and testicular veins. Ideally, you want to masturbate while lying down. See

Chapter 3: Lifestyle Changes for more details.

Scrotal Tuck: I highly recommend that you perform this exercise while lying down, before bed or with your legs up on the wall, to minimize the pressure accompanied by exercise. To get the feel for the exercise, begin by contracting your anus muscle as if you are holding back a bowel movement, or simply perform a kegel. As you do this, try to feel as if you are pulling your testicles up and toward your body. With experience, you will become more and more able to tense only your scrotal muscles. Hold the tension for a few seconds and then slowly release the muscle. It is important to have high time under tension with little rest, since the cremaster muscle is a smooth muscle that requires long time under tension to strengthen.

Like any exercise, this may not be easy to do at first and you might be able to only tighten the muscle for a moment, but aim to have the muscle under at least 1-2 minutes of tension total. You want to hold the tension for either 5 or 10 seconds and then slowly release. Rest for 1 second, and then repeat (contract and release) until you have a total time under tension of 1-2 minutes (e.g., repeat 6-12 times if you are holding the tension for 10 seconds). Perform this exercise every day before bed.

LOWER ABDOMINAL BELT

Lower abdominal belt

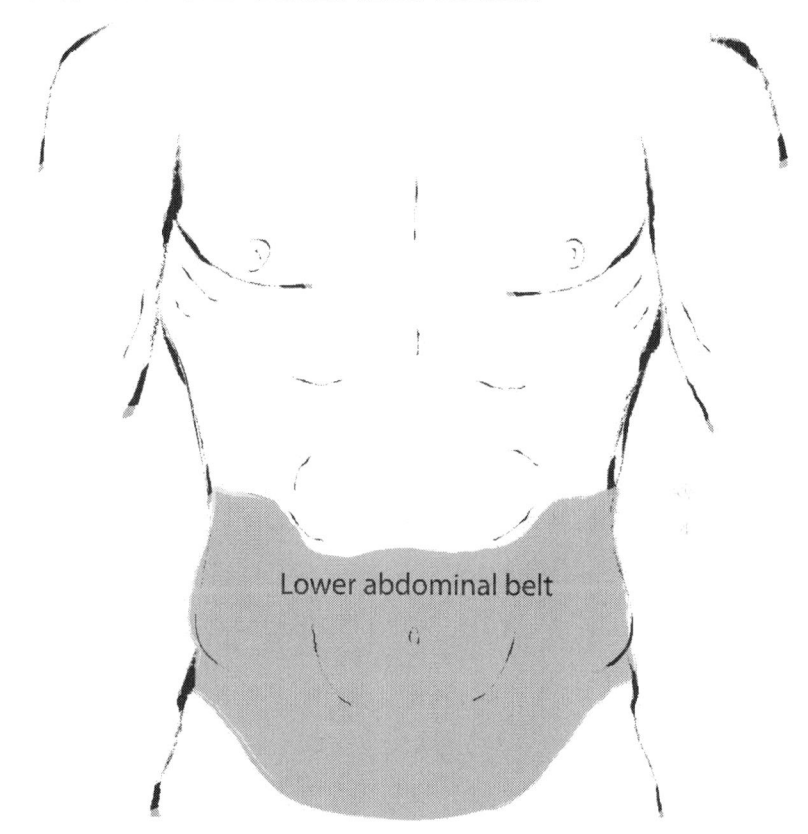

Flexing and activating your lower abs is critically important for everyone with varicocele. It helps improve blood circulation, alleviate flatulence, stimulate bowel movement, tone the lower abdominal organs, and most importantly, helps improve the tone of the abdominal belt.

The lower abdominal belt plays a critical role in minimizing pressure in the lower torso and is therefore important to strengthen and tone for long-term treatment of varicocele. You should tone your lower abdominal belt whether you spend many hours sitting or if you are very active. It will help reduce the pressure placed onto the varicocele during both sitting and physical exertion.

This is a difficult exercise to learn but is worth taking the time to learn.

Step 1: You may not know how to flex your abs. The easiest way to learn is to put your arms over your head and exhale fully. Then exhale a bit more. And a bit more! And hold. This is what flexing your abs feel like. After you really get the feel for it, try to flex your abs without this aid.

Step 2: Place your palms on your lower abs and pull in your abs. Try to focus on pulling in only your lower abs.

Step 3: While standing in front of a mirror, with your palms on your lower abs, pull in only your lower abs and then flex your abs.

Step 4: Try only flexing only your lower abs without the mirror and then without your palms on your abs.

Step 5: Flex your lower abs several times throughout the day, and when sitting, standing, or walking.

SEEK PROFESSIONAL HELP

There is a lot of value in seeking help. Many of my clients have greatly benefitted from seeking other professional help. If you are stuck and not getting good results you have the option of either contacting me or finding a specialist to help you.

Nutritionist / Dietitian: If you are making a significant change in your diet, or want advice on how to improve your weight, consult either a nutritionist or dietitian.

Fertility Specialist & General Practitioner: For pregnancy help and strategies and infertility issues, visit a fertility specialist or your general practitioner.

Personal Trainer / Physiotherapist: See a personal trainer or physiotherapist for any issues regarding posture, joint pain, muscle imbalances, and exercise technique.

General Practitioner: Visit your general practitioner regarding issues related to circulation, digestion, immune function, help quitting smoking/drinking, and any other issues.

CHAPTER DEFINITIONS

Abdominal/Diaphragm Breathing: Inhaling and exhaling with the stomach moving out and in, respectively.

Healing State: A state that allows the body to rest, heal, and digest.

Kegel: Repetitive contraction of the pelvic floor muscle.

Lower Abdominal Bet: The set of muscles and connective tissue that warp around, support, and tighten the lower abdomen.

Pelvic Floor Muscle: Muscles that help control and support the bladder and bowel.

CHAPTER 8

THE FUNDAMENTALS

These are the fundamentals that you must perform every day. The fundamentals are beneficial for almost everyone with varicocele. Practice the fundamentals alongside the treatments recommend in this guide, and I promise you that you will attain amazing results.

Remember: A combination of many treatments will get you the best results. Simply sitting in an inversion all night will not get you amazing results. Instead, for example, try keeping your testicles cool throughout the day, sitting in an inversion for 20 minutes at night, changing your diet, and improving your posture, etc.

THE FUNDAMENTALS

Fundamental 1: You must start by reading over the entire guide and applying the treatments that are relevant for you.

Fundamental 2: For the first two months of your treatment, perform minimum five cooling treatments per week.

Fundamental 3: For the first two months of your treatment, perform minimum 15 minutes of inversions daily.

Fundamental 4: Find a way to comfortably drain/improve your testicular blood circulation overnight (e.g. by elevating your hips with a pillow, keeping your testicles cool throughout the night, etc.)

Fundamental 5: Minimize excessive abdominal pressure when possible.

Fundamental 6: Keep your testicles well ventilated and cool throughout the day and at night.

Fundamental 7: After sex/masturbation, or any activity that is stressful on your varicocele/testicles, perform a cooling treatment and lay down (or perform an inversion) for minimum 5-10 minutes.

FINAL WORDS

Congratulations on picking natural treatments over varicocele surgery. I hope that you, too, now realize that varicocele is not the scary genetic disorder that mandates surgery.

Surgery is ineffective for varicocele treatment and comes with high risks. You must ask yourself: If the problem is poor blood circulation, then does it make sense to cut the veins that drain the testicles? It doesn't make sense. That is why varicocele surgery is banned in some countries and is generally not advised.

Let's look at the benefits of surgery: Only 14% improvement in pregnancy rates, along with a large body of conflicting scientific evidence? Only mild improvements in fertility, seen only in some? No significant reduction in pain symptoms? Little to no testicular size restoration after surgery? Something is wrong with this picture, especially when you add the associated risks and the high chance of reoccurrence after surgery (5-20%). Varicocele surgery is more of an aesthetic procedure that is made to look like a cure due to conflict of interest.

On the other hand, we have the best natural treatments for varicocele here. These treatments are different from surgery because they address the root cause of varicocele. Everyone should know the treatments in this guide! If we had access to this information when we were young, likely, only a few of us would have developed varicocele. Learning proper testicular care, risk-management practices, and how managing our health within the modern lifestyle is critical. I encourage everyone to teach the health practices of this guide to their children.

Please feel free to contact me at any time if you require assistance. I am here to help: daniel@varicocelehealing.com. You can also visit my website to explore the additional resources that I offer: varicocelehealing.com.

DANIEL JOHNSON

GLOSSARY

Abdominal/Diaphragm Breathing: Inhaling and exhaling with the stomach moving out and in, respectively.

Anterior Pelvic Tilt: Hip tilting forward.

Anti-Inflammatory: Chemicals or treatments that reduce inflammation.

Antioxidants: Chemicals that disable oxidants.

Arteries: Carry oxygenated blood (from lungs to heart and from heart to bodily tissues)

Body Mass Index (BMI): A simple method of categorizing people's weight relative to their height. The formula is weight in kilograms divided by height in meters squared.

Bowel Movement: The act of defecating.

Bowels: All of the digestive organs in the abdominal region.

Cremaster Muscle: The muscle of that wraps around the testicles.

Cremaster Reflex: The cremaster muscle contracts and pulls the testicles up when cold, exercising, or erect.

Defecate: Discharge feces from the body.

Epididymis: A lump on your testicles that supports sperm development.

Epididymitis: Swelling of the epididymis.

Flaccid: When the penis is soft and limp.

Forward Head Posture: The head being too far forward. It strains the entire length of the spine and pulls it out of optimal alignment.

Genital Heat Stress: Stress and damage caused by elevated scrotal/testicular temperature.

Girth: The circumference or thickness of the penis.

Glutes: The main butt muscle.

Grade I Varicocele: The varicocele is only palpable during or after Valsalva maneuver.

Grade II Varicocele: The varicocele is palpable without Valsalva maneuver.

Grade III Varicocele: The varicocele is normally visible through skin to the eyes (seen as a "bag of worms").

Hamstrings: The main muscles at the back of the thighs.

Healing State: A state that allows the body to rest, heal, and digest.

Hip Flexors: Any muscle that lips your thighs up.

Hyperthermia: Too much heat, or over-heating.

Hypothermia: Too little heat, or over-cooling.

Inflammation: A condition where a part of the body becomes red, swollen, hot, and often painful.

Intra-Abdominal Pressure: The pressure that is inside your torso. You want to minimize and manage this pressure.

Kegel: Repetitive contraction of the pelvic floor muscle.

Lower Abdominal Bet: The set of muscles and connective tissue that warp around, support, and tighten the lower abdomen.

Lymph: A clear-to-white fluid that forms in bodily tissue.

Lymphatic System: A network of vessels that have functions for the immune system and fluid retention.

Muscle Imbalance: When muscles on one side of a joint are too strong when compared to the muscles on the opposing side.

Normal Testicular Temperature: Testicular temperature when adequate heat exchange and circulation are allowed (34-36°C/93.5-96.5°F).

Note that, though very rare, a subclinical varicocele can still cause severe symptoms (normally, higher grades have more severe symptoms).

Oxidants and Reactive Oxygen Species (ROS): Chemicals that are harmful for sperm and fertility.

Pampiniform Plexus (Veins): Veins that drain from the testicles. They also function to cool the testicles.

Pelvic Floor Muscle: Muscles that help control and support the bladder and bowel.

Pelvic Tilt: The direction the hip tilts; forward or backward.

Pelvis: The hip bone.

Penis Enlargement (PE) Exercises: Any exercise, stretch, or treatment that is aimed to enlarge the penis or testicles.

Perineum: The region from the pubic bone and anus that is between the legs.

Posterior Pelvic Tilt: Hip tilting backward.

Probiotic: Any microorganism that has beneficial qualities for the body.

Quadriceps: The main muscles at the front of the thighs.

Rectus Abdominis: The six-pack muscle.

Rectus Femoris: The quadriceps muscle that also flexes the hips.

Reflux: Backflow (flow in the wrong direction) of blood.

Self-Acupressure: Pressing into specific areas with your fingers to stimulate blood flow and therapeutic effects.

Stool: Feces.

Stress: Anything that resists your being exerts stress on your system.

Subclinical Varicocele: Ultrasound analysis but not physical exam detects the presence of a varicocele.

Testicular Shrinkage/Atrophy: A condition where the testicle reduces in size.

Testis: A single testicle (singular)

Transit Time: The amount of time it takes for food to pass through the digestive system and be excreted.

Urethra: The duct through which you urinate.

Valves: To force blood to continue circulating, veins have one directional valves that prevent blood from flowing backwards.

Varicocele: Enlarged testicular veins. More specifically, it refers to the enlargement of the pampiniform plexus (veins).

Varicose Veins: Enlarged veins (general).

Vasculoprotective Agent: A substance that protects the veins from damage.

Vein Contractility: The ability of the veins to squeeze and become thinner.

Veins: Carry de-oxygenated blood (from heart to lungs and from bodily tissues back to heart)

Venous Insufficiency: Inability for veins to circulate blood.

Venous Tonifying Agent: A substance that improves vein health, energy and strength.

Printed in Great Britain
by Amazon